Self-hypnosis for health, weight loss and getting fit.

By: Kim Reader.
Bachelor of Education. Certified Hypnotherapist.

Table of Contents

Foreword

You may have purchased this book because you have tried to lose weight but have found time and time again that you have been unable to change. Maybe buying this book was a last-ditch effort to try something new to help you do something that seems so hard.

This book will take you on a journey of learning and change, which may surprise you.

Keep an open mind, some of the things you learn may be new, but if you are willing to work with the new techniques you find here, your life will change, and you will understand how to create new realities for yourself.

A Word of Caution

Self-hypnosis requires focus and is done with your eyes closed. To help you achieve your desired results, and to do so safely, you cannot engage in self-hypnosis while driving, operating equipment, caring for children, or doing anything that would require your eyes to be open and which requires your full attention.

Introduction

Each person has their own reasons for trying to lose weight and get in shape. Take a moment now to think about yours. Maybe you are concerned about your health. Perhaps you have high cholesterol, or you are worried about your heart. You may be thinking about the example you are setting for your children. Perhaps you want to feel better about how you look in your clothes and feel more confident about yourself.

Whatever your reasons, I congratulate you because by buying this book and learning how to use self-hypnosis, you will lose all the weight you choose to, keep it off for the rest of your life, and feel fantastic while doing it.

There are a few things for you to understand about this process before getting started. It is important that you understand these concepts, because they will enable you to get the full effect of your program of self-hypnosis.

Understanding your mind

You may not think much about how your mind works. You may find it interesting to learn that your mind is separated into separate and distinct parts. Each section is responsible for different things and they sometimes have the difficulty of having competing ideas about how we should think and behave.

Having competing ideas can, of course, make it difficult to make changes to our behaviour. Let's take a moment to learn about how the mind works because, for you to achieve change in your life it is important to understand something about how your mind works. For the purposes of weight loss, we will focus on understanding the conscious and subconscious parts of your mind.

The conscious mind

The conscious part of your mind is the part of your mind that is at work when you are driving a car or walking or talking. That is the level you are at right now and it is the part of the mind where we spend most of our time. The conscious mind has four main functions.

Its first job is to **analyze**. It looks at problems, reviews them and comes up with a decision as to how to solve the problem. It is the part of the mind that makes all the decisions that need to be made daily like; what to wear, what time to get up and all of the other small and large decisions we make each day. Decisions such as should I open the door, may seem automatic, but are in fact choices made by our conscious mind.

The part of our conscious mind that can be the part that gets us in trouble when we want to make changes to our habit is called the **rational** mind. This part of the mind provides us with rational reasons for our behaviour. For example, a smoker may tell themselves things such as, "I smoke because it makes me feel calm and gives me time to gather my thoughts." Or an overweight person may say "I eat because I am nervous or bored", or because it is hereditary.

These reasons provided by the rational part of our conscious mind are never original and these reasons often come from others. An overweight person may have heard these comments from family or friends and after hearing statements like these so many times, they adopt them as their own reasons for continuing a behaviour that they know is harmful to them.

The next part of the conscious mind is the **willpower**, which is something I think most people who have tried to lose weight are familiar with. Willpower is what we are relying upon, when we wake up in the morning and say to ourselves. "Today is the day I am going to completely give up junk food." Usually, our willpower gives out by the end of the day, and when our willpower weakens, the old pattern returns. Relying on willpower and failing repeatedly, can actually make us feel worse and can make it seem like we cannot change. Willpower is usually not enough to help a person change a habit.

The last part of the conscious mind is what we call the **working memory**. This is the memory that we need to function every day. Questions like "What is the best way to get to work today?", or "What am I going to need to take for my trip on the weekend?" are both questions that are answered by the information stored in the working memory.

The analytical mind, the rational mind, the willpower and the working memory are all parts of the conscious mind. Think about Spock from television when envisioning the conscious mind. Like this famous character, our conscious mind can only behave in an analytical way. Changing habits like improving our diet and beginning an exercise regime requires far more than the conscious mind can provide.

The subconscious mind

Below the conscious mind is the subconscious mind. While the conscious mind is logical and rational, the subconscious mind is the emotional part of the mind. It is additionally responsible for recording and storing all the experiences that we have had throughout our lives. This information comes from the lessons taught to us by our parents, from teachers, and from the world we live in. This information becomes the programming that guides our opinions, beliefs and behaviours. This includes our opinions, beliefs, and behaviours relates to losing weight and exercise.

From an extremely early age, we have learned many lessons taught to us by the numerous experiences we have had. These lessons have a powerful impact upon us. Our subconscious mind is like a computer and stores these experiences, and just like a computer it has no choice but to respond to the programming contained there. Whatever is programmed there must come true.

This is vitally important. You may have heard about the self-fulfilling prophecy. This prophecy points to the fact that if you believe something you behave in a way that guarantees that it comes true. For example, if you are trying to reduce your weight, but your subconscious programming holds the belief that you have never been able to lose weight, so this time will be no different, it is extremely unlikely that you will have success. That is because you will behave in a way that confirms your belief that you will fail.

Think for a moment about all the beliefs about eating, or food or exercise that have been programmed into your own subconscious mind. Maybe you were told to clean your plate even when you were no longer hungry. Perhaps you were heavy as a child and were told you would be overweight all of your life. These experiences become part of your belief system. As an adult you may rationally think all of the things you heard from parents and caregivers may be silly, but despite rationally knowing these beliefs aren't true, this subconscious baggage still controls how you behave and may be the reason reaching weight loss goals are so difficult.

This type of programming is what drives many people to overeat. They simply cannot act in any other way because their programming tells them to act that way. When we look at how this works while keeping the self-fulfilling prophecy in mind, it becomes obvious that if we believe at the subconscious level that we are destined to be overweight, we will be unable to take off weight.

This programming is extremely powerful and it is the reason that willpower is not strong enough for most people to create changes to their habits. Willpower is just not enough. Willpower may work for a short period of time, but it is usually overridden by that strong, powerful information about how who you are, and how you are meant to operate, which is stored in the subconscious mind.

The good news is that the programming in the subconscious mind can change. It often changes in a natural way. As we have new experiences, our perspectives about ourselves and the world can be changed by new information. For example, if you if you were bitten by a dog, it may create a long-standing belief that dogs are dangerous. However, if later in your life you get to know somebody who owns a dog, and you spend time around it, you may begin to feel comfortable around the dog. Slowly the fear you have begins to change, and your negative feelings towards dogs are replaced with more favourable programming. Over time the happy and positive experiences build and eventually you feel completely comfortable around dogs.

This is a simple explanation of how the programming of the subconscious mind can be changed. **Beliefs can also be changed in a more direct way by using self-hypnosis.**

Many people try to lose weight, eat better and exercise more. Many of these new goals begin with a New Year's resolution which follows a Christmas time blow out of too much food and drink. It is unfortunate that many people who try to make these important health changes fail within days or weeks. Regardless of what time of the year you were unsuccessful in losing the extra weight you have been carrying, changes need to be made. There are many reasons for failure, but chief amongst them is an inability to change your long-standing beliefs about whether you can be successful. If we cannot make changes to our beliefs, changing our habits will be virtually impossible.

Habits are difficult to overcome because for many of us, our habits have been with us for years, and likely for decades. Some people have been "on a diet for years." These habits may also be very ingrained in our subconscious minds because we learned early in life from our families, and because of this, we may be completely at a loss as to how to give these habits up. There is also the additional problem that people who want to begin to eat more healthily, or who want to exercise, may also have the difficulty of not knowing what it means to have healthy habits.

This book can help you with these challenges and others.

Chapter 1

How Does One Change Their Beliefs and Habits?

Beliefs which are the basis of habits, can be changed by replacing them with new more positive beliefs. Many people have beliefs that keep them stuck. They have beliefs that have been with them so long they have become part of their subconscious programming about themselves and they become obstacles that may seem impossible to overcome. The good news is that subconscious programming can be changed. Self-hypnosis is one of the best ways to change your beliefs.

The history of hypnosis

You may have heard about hypnosis and the many forms it takes. Hypnosis can be used by a skillful stage hypnotist to create an amazing show that has some audience members engaged in jaw dropping stunts, where they seemingly have no control over their body or their mind. Stage hypnotism has been around for hundreds of years and has astounded audiences for just as long.

Stage hypnosis shows are just one part of the numerous ways hypnosis can be used. Hypnosis in the form of visualization, laying on of hands, and meditation has been used in one way or another for centuries to help suffers of all types of pain and illness get relief in many parts of the world.

An early believer and practitioner of hypnosis was Franz Anton Mesmer. Dr. Mesmer was born in Germany and published a book called, *Mesmerism: The Discovery of Animal Magnetism* in 1779. Dr. Mesmer discovered that changes could be brought about in the health of his patients by sitting close to them and holding their hands sometimes for hours.

Dr. Mesmer saw many patients and gave many demonstrations of his powers. He became famous throughout Europe and became famous for his ability to cure a variety of physical and emotional ailments. At the time Dr. Mesmer attributed his success to something he called "animal magnetism."

Modern reflection upon the doctor's ability to cure his patients, asserts that his fame, social standing and the belief by his patients that he could cure them, were significant contributors to his success. This concept holds true today. The things we believe to be true are the things that happen for us. The word "mesmerize", which means to cause somebody to act as though they are under a spell, comes from Dr. Mesmer's name is often used interchangeably with the word "hypnosis".

Dr. James Braid, a Scottish surgeon, born in 1795, became fascinated by Anton Mesmer while viewing one of Mesmer's stage performances where he cured a variety of ailments for his audience. Braid initially viewed Mesmer as some kind of a con-artist, and his intent in studying Mesmer, was initially to discredit him and to prove that Mesmer's powers were nothing more than fraud.

Dr. Braid soon realized that, Mesmer's success with his subjects were due to the power of the man himself and his subject's willingness to allow themselves to visualize their own healing. What was true in Mesmer's time holds true today, the power of hypnosis to heal is dependent upon the skills of the hypnotist and the willingness of the subject to accept the suggestions the hypnotist provides.

Dr. Braid was in fact the first person to describe the instructions Dr. Mesmer gave his subjects as "suggestions." He was also the first person to describe Dr. Mesmer's techniques as "hypnosis." This term was based upon the Greek word for sleep, "hypnos." This word is still used today to describe all forms of hypnosis despite the fact that hypnosis and sleep are completely different.

Hypnotism continues to be used in a clinical setting to help clients overcome problems such as smoking, overeating or to overcome stress. A skilled practitioner uses their knowledge and skills to help clients determine why they have not been able to give up habits they may have tried to kick numerous times without success.

The practitioner then creates suggestions which are simply instructions which help change subconscious programming so old beliefs can be discarded and the client can overcome their negative habits. If the client's goal is to let go of weight, their weight loss goal can be made to be become their number one priority and the client can be helped to have control over what they eat and the amount of exercise they are getting.

What is hypnosis?

Stage hypnotism, and clinical hypnotism share several important attributes and understanding how they work is important. In each case a subject is placed into a hypnotic state which is achieved by having the client listen to suggestions from the hypnotist. The hypnotized state is simply a deep state of relaxation. Reaching the hypnotic state is important because the hypnotic state enables the hypnotist to give suggestions to the subject's subconscious mind.

A suggestion is an instruction which the subject chooses to accept, and which can cause them to put on a great show for a stage hypnotist or make changes to their habits in the case of clinical hypnosis.

The hypnotic state feels very relaxing, and is sometimes confused with sleep. However, sleep, and the deeply relaxed state are quite different. This deeply relaxed state enables the subject to become very focused on the instructions (suggestions) given to them by the hypnotist.

In this state the mind is relaxed, yet open and willing to accept the suggestions, which are beneficial and crafted to help the subject make changes to their subconscious programming. The hypnotic state looks from the outside much like sleep and in fact the word sleep is often used by the hypnotist to induce a state where the subconscious mind can be reached, and suggestions can be accepted.

While the subject or client is in a hypnotic state, they feel very drowsy and relaxed. The subject may in fact feel quite sleepy. The mind is peaceful and relaxed and clear of outside thoughts. However, unlike sleep the mind is in an active state and the hypnotist can be heard.

Reaching this state of "wakeful sleep" is very important. When you are in this state the conscious part of the mind is at rest. Reaching this state is also important because the conscious mind tends to be skeptical and will block the new positive suggestions the hypnotherapist is sharing with the client. When the hypnotic state is reached a clinical hypnotherapist, or stage hypnotist can give suggestions which can by-pass the conscious mind and reach the subconscious mind.

If you have ever been to a stage hypnosis show, then you know that some people do not become part of the performance. During a hypnosis show, a stage hypnotist will typically start by asking audience members questions such as "who enjoys having fun?" or "Who wants to be part of a great show?" Some people will keep their hands firmly tucked in their pockets, not wanting to risk being hypnotized by mistake. Other audience members will jump up and down while screaming, "Me, me, pick me!" The hypnotist will choose these enthusiastic members of the audience and welcome them onto the stage and confirm their suitability to be in the show by giving some basic suggestions to see if they are as ready to be hypnotized as they appear. If the simple suggestions are readily accepted by the subject they will stay on the stage, while those who do not accept the suggestions will be thanked for their time and be asked to return to their seats.

The people who remain on the stage have decided to begin a journey with the hypnotist.

Similarly, clients in a clinical hypnotherapist's office must be willing to accept the suggestions given to them by their hypnotherapist.

After determining what issues will be addressed in the hypnosis session, a hypnotherapist will typically begin a session by asking their client to relax, get comfortable, and close their eyes. Sitting in a comfortable chair with the lights low is an ideal setting. The hypnotherapist will then ask the client to allow their mind to relax as much as possible and to allow their mind to accept the positive suggestions they are going to hear.

The client and hypnotherapist are equals on this journey. While the hypnotherapist may have experience and skill in the techniques of hypnosis, the client must decide they will accept the suggestions given to them. Without cooperation between the hypnotherapist and client, the best hypnotherapist in the world will be unable to help their client make the changes they want.

Reaching a deeply relaxed is crucial because it is in this state that the suggestions of the hypnotherapist can bypass the skeptical conscious mind and be accepted as new programming by the subconscious mind.

Like the members of the audience in the stage hypnosis show, clients in the hypnotherapy office must be willing to accept the new programming given in the form of suggestions. Suggestions cannot be forced into a client's subconscious mind. Likewise, when you begin to use self-hypnosis to change your own beliefs and habits, the suggestions you give your subconscious mind must be accepted and are not something that can be forced.

Some people have asked me if a hypnotist can make a person do things that they would not do if they were fully awake. The answer to this question is an emphatic "no". The subconscious mind cannot be programmed in that manner. Keep in mind that the subject is awake during hypnosis, just in a very relaxed state. At any time, a client can open their eyes, and end their session.

Hypnotic suggestions need to be positive and must be accepted by the client. If a client was given a suggestion that went against their morals or made them uncomfortable in any way, the suggestion would be rejected, and the client could simply leave the session.

There is no need to worry if hypnosis
can make you do something that you are uncomfortable with,
hypnosis simply does not work that way. The client and the
hypnotist are equals and must work together to have a
successful hypnosis session. You are perfectly safe and in
control the whole time you are involved in hypnosis.

Chapter 2

Emily's Weight Loss Story

Emily is a 32-year-old teacher. On her first visit to my office, she was feeling tired, and she stated that it seemed like she had less and less energy to devote to working with her students. She also reported that she often felt grouchy while she was with them. She also said that she had no energy to exercise or socialize after work, which was making her feel unhappy with her life. She hated that her clothing felt tight, and she told me that she wanted to lose 30 pounds.

Emily explained that she began gaining weight when she got her teaching job, 10 years earlier. Teaching kept her very busy and it felt like she had no time to cook healthy dinners or prepare healthy lunches. She typically stopped for coffee and a donut on the way to school and went out at lunch for more fast food.

Emily described her life to me, and it was clear that she is a devoted teacher. Her evenings and weekends are filled with preparing lessons and marking her student's work. She didn't want to take time to shop for nutritious food and often relied on ordering pizza or other food so she would not have to cook. She described how much work she felt she had to do to keep up and she admitted she felt guilty if she took a bit of time for herself to go shopping for healthy food, or to take a break to get some exercise. She felt more and more sluggish and without noticing, she began to become less physically active. In fact, she eventually got to the point where she got almost no exercise at all. She felt that she had really lost control of her own body and to a great extent she had given up on even trying.

While discussing Emily's difficulties in losing weight, she disclosed that her parents and several of her aunts and uncles were overweight, and that she had lately begun to wonder if she was just like them. Emily had a close relationship with her mother, and throughout Emily's life, the two had had, numerous conversations about weight loss, dieting and exercise.

In our initial conversation about Emily's background and childhood, it was clear that Emily's mother had many of the same beliefs, feelings and problems as Emily. For example, they both believed that preparing healthy meals and lunches would take up too much time, and that it was simpler to buy fast food. They each believed that they were too busy to get out for a walk or bike ride and that the gym was too scary. They were both approximately 30 pounds overweight, and they both felt sluggish. They had each been on numerous diets and had little success with reducing their weight. Neither one of them had any idea where to start to release the extra weight they had been carrying.

Their lack of success had left each of them with negative feelings about their ability to make changes. Emily's mom had tried every type of diet over the course of many years and her experiences impacted Emily in a negative way. When Emily was growing up, she watched as her mom struggled, lost weight and then re-gained it. Emily also became somebody that her mother talked to about her weight loss struggles. This of course, helped shape Emily's ideas about weight loss and she grew up believing that weight loss was impossible.

Children learn from listening to their parents and are like sponges who are always soaking in knowledge about their world by watching their parent's behaviour. Watching what had happened to her mom had left Emily with real doubts that she could be successful. Her mother also told Emily on numerous occasions that Emily was built like her, that she got the bad genes from her side of the family, and that losing weight was the hardest thing in the world. Comments such as these coming from a major role model became the subconscious programming Emily had to overcome in order to change her life.

Now that Emily was an adult, she retained all these beliefs about herself that she learned early in her life. There was no chance of Emily losing weight when deep down, she had no reason to believe that she would be successful. This makes sense because our subconscious programming is very powerful and overrides our willpower.

Emily wanted to lose weight, but with programming telling her that she was destined to fail, she had very little chance of success. Even when we have a goal, when the programming stored in the subconscious mind is not supportive of that goal, failure will be likely. People may attempt to use willpower and think that willpower alone will enable them to be successful. This is just is not the case.

The subconscious mind is charge of your behaviour and if it doesn't change then you cannot make the changes you desperately want to make. Emily's programming was clear, she was destined to fail because she had bad genes, she had the same problems as her mother, and like her mother had said time and time again, "losing weight is impossible." Her mother's negative experiences had left Emily wanting to lose weight but with very little chance of being successful.

How hypnosis helped Emily

It was obvious to me when I spoke to Emily, that she had many beliefs about healthy eating and exercise that were getting in her way. Emily was unclear about why she couldn't lose weight and had never thought about an important fact that we all must accept if we want to make changes to our lives. The truth of the matter is this; if we continue to believe at the subconscious level that we will fail, then we will fail. If we change our thoughts at the subconscious level to "I succeed" then we can successfully make changes to our habits.

There is no chance of losing weight if you believe at the subconscious level that you have no chance of being successful. Negative beliefs must be addressed and changed to positive beliefs. Self-hypnosis is one of the easiest ways to influence the subconscious mind.

During our first session, Emily was asked to keep track of any negative thoughts she had about losing weight and getting healthy, in a journal. As she recorded her negative self-talk, it became clear to her that she had a very negative attitude towards succeeding in her goals to lose weight and become more physically fit.

She recorded numerous instances each day when she thought in a negative way about whether she could successfully lose weight and get in shapes. She recorded the negative thoughts and realized these thoughts sounded exactly like the things her mom had said over and over again when discussing her own battle to reduce her weight.

Emily, like many other clients, was surprised about how many times she reinforced her own negative thoughts each day and understood clearly how hard it would be to lose weight with so much negative thinking.

Emily realized quickly in part, because she had often explained the exact same way of thinking to her young students. She had often reminded students who were struggling to learn, that they needed to keep a positive attitude and to refrain from using phrases such as "I will never learn to write better," or "I hate math'" or "I suck at math." Emily instinctively knew that her students had to change their beliefs in order to be a success at school. She also began to realize that her own thinking about weight loss was making it impossible for her to change.

Emily's negative beliefs and self-talk included

I am too busy to lose weight.
I am too busy to cook and prepare healthy food.
I am too busy to exercise.
People in my family cannot lose weight.
I will fail, so why even try.
I don't care if I am overweight.
People in my family always give up when trying to lose weight.
Losing weight is too hard.
I have to use all my time to work on being a great teacher.

These beliefs, and negative self-talk were responsible for Emily's inability to lose weight. It makes sense. If you think you will fail to lose weight, it is not very likely that you will be able to change the habits which are making you overweight. I know this may seem obvious, but time and time again, I have worked with people who are desperate to lose weight and can't understand why they can't make it happen.

How athletes use self-hypnosis to improve athletic performance

Take a moment to think about successful athletes. You may be surprised to learn that world-class athletes practice self-hypnosis and visualization of their ability to hit better or run faster. What result would a marathon runner have, if each day before starting their training they said to themselves, "I will never improve". Or "My parents couldn't run fast, so neither can I." Or "Everybody else is better so I might as well give up."

Can you see in this example how pointless it would be for the athlete to even bother to train? The athlete would clearly fail to improve. In fact, I doubt that an athlete with those beliefs would continue to practice. There would be no purpose. They would be too unmotivated to even try. In fact, coaches and top athletes believe strongly in the benefit of positive suggestions and many make use of self-hypnosis daily as part of their training routines. They know how important it is that their mind leads the way to their body's ability to break world records.

Top athletes typically spend time each day, reaching a deep relaxed state where they repeat positive affirmations and visualization of all the ways that their athletic performance will improve. This has become quite standard in sports programs from college football teams to the NBA. The reason leading athletes use these techniques is because they have been found to work. They can work for any aspect of our life including to help us lose weight and get fit.

In terms of being successful, you are no different than the athlete described above. An athlete cannot succeed while continuing to doubt themselves and neither can you. An athlete who continues to repeat negative self-talk, will never get faster. In fact, the athlete would probably give up on their training. Similarly, for weight loss to occur, for you, changes to your beliefs must be made. Without the belief that you can be successful, it is very unlikely that you can be successful in reaching your weight loss goal. It would also be very likely that you would not even try.

This book will help you understand how your own thoughts and feelings have become your beliefs, and how they have solidified into your habits. This book will help you understand how they have blocked you from moving forward to overcome negativity so that the changes you have wanted can take place.

Your subconscious mind is similar in many ways to the hard drive in a computer. It is always running in the background, and it controls what happens although we are unaware of what it is doing. Like a computer, the subconscious mind has an operating system which is filled with commands. A computer's hard drive consists of the programming it uses to run all the systems needed to make the computer run efficiently. Our subconscious mind has all the programming required to run you.

This is exactly the way the sub-conscious mind operates. It functions much like a computer, however it is much more powerful. We program our mind's subconscious computer everyday through our life experiences.

While a computer has programming that has been loaded by a programmer, our subconscious mind also has programming which has been loaded in by other people. Our parents, teachers, and caregivers of all kinds have an impact on how we think about ourselves. Messages from the media also contribute to our beliefs. The programming found in this part of the mind, is placed there daily, year after year, and decade after decade, and determines what we come to believe is true about ourselves. Here is an example of how programming becomes part of your subconscious programming, and how it shapes your daily life.

Clients sometimes seek help to overcome a fear of public speaking. This is a common fear and for some people overcoming it becomes necessary due to a job change, an upcoming wedding or other necessary social commitments. Some people admit they have "always hated public speaking" and would not be seeking help unless life changes or special events hadn't come along to make it necessary.

This common fear can be typically be traced back to certain experiences in which the client felt nervous, anxious, and perhaps humiliated. The experience was upsetting and created a great deal of negative programming. This negative programming becomes part of the clients operating system. The client's fear often becomes worse over the years as the client tries to avoid public speaking and hears the comments from friends and family about the terrors of speaking in front of a crowd.

Typical subconscious programming found in clients with a fear of public speaking:

- Memories of being forced as children to make a speech or presentation in school which left the child with feelings of terror and a sense of being humiliated.

- Feelings of embarrassment about the speech or presentation which lead to a dread of being forced to have to do it again sometime in the future.

- Negative self-talk such as "I am a terrible public speaker" or "I hate public speaking." The negative feelings lead to a lack of confidence or perhaps a fear of getting into situations where they may have to speak in front of others.

- Reinforcement of negative feelings by others. For example, "Public speaking is the worst "or "I hate public speaking too."

- Feeling "dumb" about how poorly their speeches have gone up until now.

- Avoidance of any kind of public speaking which serves to reinforce negative feelings about themselves.

The subconscious programming described above is typical for clients with the fear of public speaking. Subconscious programming exists for every habit a client wants to overcome. For most negative habits you may have, the programming has existed for years, and maybe decades, and has been reinforced in your subconscious mind many thousands of times. The negative reinforcement is internal (your own feelings of fear repeated). As mentioned above, negative reinforcement can come from external forces as well.

Here is an example of how outside forces can impact your subconscious programming. You speak to a friend about an upcoming speech you must make. The friend agrees with you that public speaking is a horrible experience. The friend does not want to harm you, but the more they agree with how upsetting the experience of public speaking can be, the more it serves to reinforce your own thoughts. It would be better for the friend to respond to your concerns by trying to encourage you and offer help instead of agreeing with you that it will be an awful experience.

One other thing to keep in mind about negative programming at the subconscious level is that the longer you have had the problem you would like to overcome, the more likely it is that you have solidified your negative feelings about whether you can successfully overcome it. Overcoming this negative programming takes change at the subconscious level.

Subconscious programming has an emotional component as well

Much of the programming found in our subconscious minds is strongly linked to our emotions and that is why it has so much power over the things we do every day. For example, when a client talks about their fear of public speaking, they often recount a terrible experience that occurred when they were young and that involved feelings of embarrassment and shame. The client when thinking of this event for years afterwards, re-experiences those feelings and in a sense, re-lives that embarrassment repeatedly.

It is not uncommon for adult clients to blush, have a stomach-ache or feel sweaty when talking about their initial experiences. These reactions show how the subconscious mind has the power to control how our body functions in addition to having control over our habits.

Think about it this way. If you feel sweaty, have pains in your stomach, feel shaky or blush at the thought of something that happened decades earlier, it shows that you must have subconscious programming that is powerful. Overcoming that programming is essential to moving forward to new beliefs and personal success.

Preparing Emily's self-hypnosis script

The following self-hypnosis script is the one that Emily and I created together. She recorded the four parts together on her cell phone so that she could listen to it more than once each day. Emily started out by listening to her script in the morning before getting out of bed, and then again in the early evening. Emily liked to listen to it before getting out of bed as it helped her focus on her goals for the day and she said it kept her programming fresh in her mind. Additionally, she liked to listen to it just after dinner, as that was the time of day when she was starting to think about her next day.

This system worked great for Emily. Some people choose to listen to their script in the morning and then right before bed. Right before bed didn't work for Emily but for many people getting into bed at night and listening to their self-hypnosis recording works best. The reason just before bed works well is because you are likely quite relaxed at that time, which quiets the skeptical conscious mind, so the new programming can reach the subconscious mind easily.

The second reason that this time of day works so well is because the new programming becomes part of your dreams.

I recommend that you repeat your script twice per day initially because it ensures that the new information works quickly to change your old programming so that new habits can take root.

If you repeat the script twice a day, you will be amazed about how different you feel, and how easy it is to be successful. I suggest you listen to your script twice per day for at least two weeks. Remember, you are working towards overcoming years or decades of negative thoughts and feelings.

The four parts of a self-hypnosis script

There are four parts to a self-hypnosis session. The four parts are called the induction, the suggestions, the post-hypnotic suggestions and emerging from hypnosis. Each session should include all 4 parts. Let's take a moment to review what is included in each part.

<u>Induction</u>

In this part of the session, you will take yourself to a very relaxed state so that your sub-conscious mind can be given the suggestions that you have created. It is important that you listen to your self-hypnosis recording more than once so that changes can be made to the programming in your subconscious mind. The conscious mind as we have discussed tends to be skeptical and by first, entering a deeply relaxed state the conscious mind can be bypassed and the subconscious mind can be reached.

There are a variety of inductions that can be used to reach a deeply relaxed state. You will find several at the back of this book. Use the one that helps you become relaxed most easily.

<u>Suggestions</u>

Suggestions are the instructions you will be giving to your subconscious mind. While presenting suggestions to the subconscious mind, they should be given in the present tense. The reason for this is because the subconscious mind responds best when information is presented in this manner. You must avoid phrases that such as "I will lose weight" or "I will be healthy." Instead use "I lose weight", or "I successfully lose weight", "I enjoy my healthy eating plan" or "exercise makes me feel so good." Form your suggestions in the present tense so the subconscious mind understands that it is something you are doing now, not sometime in the future.

Suggestions that were used by clients discussed in this book, can be used by you to help with your own goals. It is recommended however that you fill in the form found in this book, so that your suggestions are personalized to help overcome your specific negative programming. Taking your time while determining your own negative beliefs is important.

The negative information you have been carrying around is after all, the reason you cannot reach your goals, so please try to think about your own negative self-talk, and the beliefs you may have been holding onto since you were young. It may take some time to come up with a full list. Perhaps you will need help from a close friend or family member. When you have you have completed your form and you feel you have successfully uncovered all of your negative beliefs, and determined all of your negative self-talk, you are ready to use the information to create your own suggestions.

Post-hypnotic suggestions

This type of suggestion gives you an additional boost to your programming between your self-hypnosis sessions. For the purposes of taking off weight they are extremely helpful because unlike smoking where a client intends to give up smoking completely, a person who wants to lose weight, still must plan what they will eat, they have to shop, they must also prepare food and eat.

Post-hypnotic suggestions are small suggestions that you place into your subconscious mind during your self-hypnosis sessions and which are cued by certain behaviors that you engage in often in the normal course of your day. When post-hypnotic suggestions are incorporated into your new programming, they serve to renew your suggestions many times per day, which is helpful in terms of successfully letting go of old habits.

Here are some examples of post-hypnotic suggestions that could be added to your self-hypnosis script.

- Each time I eat food I notice that I find I feel full and satisfied more quickly and that I find the feeling of being really stuffed with food unpleasant.

- Each time I pick up my fork, I remember the phrase "I eat slowly" and I repeat the phrase three times in my mind, and I notice I eat my food more slowly and I feel full and satisfied more quickly.

- Each time I think about the gym, I think about how good I feel after I exercise, and I know I want this experience this feeling again and again. Each time I go to the gym I feel proud, energized and motivated.

- Each time I look at a calendar, I think of that date in the future that I have circled on the calendar. I think of that special date in the future when I have reached my weight loss and fitness goal.

- Each morning when I brush my teeth, I feel energized and motivated to reach my weight loss goal and I am convinced I can succeed.

Re-emergence

This part of your self-hypnosis program is the part where you come out of your deep relaxed state. It is important to take some time to re-emerge because you will likely feel sleepy and relaxed and you want to ensure you are fully wide awake before you continue with your day. Do not skip this important step, or you may feel groggy for a few minutes afterwards.

Emily's self-hypnosis script

To follow is the script Emily used to take off her weight. She recorded it on her phone and listened to it in the morning and in the early evening. I have included all four parts: The induction, the suggestions, the post-hypnotic suggestions and the re-emergence. You must include all four parts and record them to create your own self-hypnosis script.

I have noted where each part begins but, when you record your own self-hypnosis script you will simply flow from one section to the next. Before listening to your self-hypnosis script, make sure you are in a warm comfortable place. You may choose to wear headphones as they will block out background noise. You will be closing your eyes, so ensure you are in a safe place where you do not have to worry about having to open your eyes part-way through your session. Obviously, these life changing sessions require your full attention and are done with your eyes closed, so please do not listen to your self-hypnosis script program while driving.

Part 1 of Emily's self-hypnosis program

<u>Induction or relaxation stage</u>

My mind is ready to listen to all the suggestions about becoming slim and healthy through new ways of eating and new programs of exercise. The suggestions here are powerful and change my body, mind and spirit. I allow myself to take in these suggestions and they enable me to become a success. People become what they believe to be true and that is why it is important to remember to think about how successful I am. Losing weight and eating the foods that will help maintain a healthy slim body is now something that I can do. I maintain my habits and the weight stays off.

I am about to allow myself to go to a deeply relaxed state where, the suggestions I hear are clear and powerful changes are made to my subconscious mind.

I imagine myself at the top of a beautiful long stone staircase. The details of the railing are beautiful, and the stone beneath my feet is smooth and I am ready to take the first step.

Looking at the staircase makes me feel relaxed and I know that as I travel down the steps, I become more relaxed with each step. I travel down the staircase and each step enables me to become ten times more relaxed. Each step takes me to a deeper state of relaxation.

Slowly, I take the first step down, and I let my relaxation deepen. It feels so good to relax and each step feels more and more relaxing.

I take the second step and I feel more comfortable more relaxed, each step making me ten times more relaxed. Third step now, more relaxed and letting go. Forth step and it feels so good just to let go, and I allow myself to go to an even more deeply relaxed state. The fifth step and I am already so relaxed, but I want to go even deeper, so I take the sixth step and it feels so good just to let go. Now the seventh step and I am close to being completely relaxed but I want to go even deeper, the more relaxed I am, the better I feel. The eighth step now and I am really enjoying this feeling. I feel dreamy and relaxed, my body is relaxed, and my mind is ready for the powerful suggestions I know will enable me to release the weight I choose to let go of. Now the ninth step, I see it and I take the step knowing how good it feels to be so relaxed. I have reached the tenth and final step and I take the step knowing I am relaxed and ready for the suggestions that change the habits I have chosen to release.

Now that I have reached the bottom of the staircase, I feel relaxed and peaceful and so ready to be a success. In this deeply relaxed state, I look around notice a mirror. It is not a regular mirror which shows how I look, but instead it is a special mirror which shows me how I look at the perfect weight for me.

I see myself at the perfect weight. I notice how my arms look, they look slim and fit. My legs look strong and they are the right size for me. They look exactly how I want them to look and I notice their shape and size, and I notice every detail and those details inspire me to be successful. I also notice my waist and my chest. These areas of my body look just the way I want them to. Slim, fit, and the muscles firm and fit. Strong and healthy.

I notice my neck and my face. My face looks younger and fit and healthy, I look so healthy and confident. My jawline is strong, and I look relaxed and happy. This is a very vivid image, and I can see it. I am so inspired to reach the perfect weight for me, and it makes it so easy to release extra weight.

My imagination is vivid, and I am so ready to receive these new and powerful suggestions. I am a success. I have been successful in so many ways. I am a great teacher, and one thing I have always said to my students is that "you can achieve anything you set your mind to." I have decided to set my mind to releasing my excess weight and starting an exercise program. I know this is the most natural thing in the world for me.

Part 2

<u>Suggestions</u>

As a successful person, I know that I can make changes, set goals and reach those goals easily. One thing I have decided to do is to eat better food. I feel great when I eat better food, and the thought of feeling even better when I teach excites me. I have researched online, and I have created an eating plan that works for me. It has a lot of variety and I know it is enjoyable.

I have even made a grocery list so that I know what to buy. I have found a way to have the groceries delivered, and I schedule it for a time when I am home marking schoolwork, so it takes no time at all. It is easy, it is efficient, and it saves me time. I love that my new way of living is actually a time saver. My new way of eating saves me time!

It is easy to maintain my new habits. I eat three healthy meals a day and I have healthy snacks too. I eat the right amount of healthy food; I feel really excited. I am healthy and energized. I eat the right amount of food, I feel satisfied. I feel strong.

This is such an easy plan, and it works so well for me. It is natural for me and the weight leaves my body easily.

I notice that this new plan saves time during the day too. I do not have to go out during the day to buy food and I notice I now have time to head out for a walk with a co-worker each day. We walk for 20 minutes and it works so well. I enjoy how my body feels, and how good my mind feels after some time outdoors. I really enjoy this time I take for myself.

It is interesting that this little bit of time makes me a better teacher. I feel energized and I have learned a lot from my co-worker. A walk outdoors gives me time to solve work challenges which makes school even easier. I notice I feel healthier and I feel cheerful and energized with the kids. It just makes sense that having a 20-minute break during the day actually saves me time because I have time to think and find ways to make my school day easier. Taking this time is so natural and so simple.

I have decided to be a success in changing my body, in the same way I have been successful in other parts of my life. It makes sense, I am a successful person, so I am successful in this part of my life too.

Family is important to me; I enjoy the time I have with them. I continue to have fun with them just like I always have. We talk, we laugh, we share our concerns, and I am still their supportive daughter and they are still my loving family. This always stays the same. I have decided that if family members want to make changes, I can give them help and support. I share this program with them, I tell them about how I have been eating.

Some may choose to join me on walks when we get together, and I really enjoy that. They can join in on my new way of life, but they may not, but I continue with what I know is right for me, and that is ok. I have control over what I eat, and how much I eat, and when I exercise. I have made a choice and I am successful. My family still loves me, and I love them.

For the first time in a long time, I have a plan, and this excites me and makes me extremely successful. I have planned out the best way for me to lose weight and so, I am a success. This seems so easy this time, I can do this. I know having a plan, is the key to releasing weight and now I know exactly how to do it. Just like I had to learn how to be a good teacher, I had to learn how to slim down and get in shape. I know how to be successful and I am a success, just like I have been in so many areas of my life. This time is so much different than other times I tried to release weight, because I know what to do and I feel confident following the plan I created.

The suggestions I give myself sink deep into my subconscious mind and change my programming. It feels good to do something that I know makes me a success.

My mind returns to the image of myself at my perfect weight. I notice how strong, healthy and happy I look. I look in the

mirror and the image is clear in my mind. This image becomes
very vivid to me and I know I am successful.

Part 3

<u>Post-hypnotic suggestions</u>

Each time before I begin to eat, the image of myself at the
perfect weight for me enters my mind. I think about it and this
image becomes strong. I can see the details of how I look at
my perfect weight, I see my face, my chest and stomach, my
hips and my arms and legs. I look healthy and fit, energetic
and young and amazing. This image helps me. It enters my
mind when I eat and I notice I feel full faster, I enjoy the
healthy foods I have chosen for myself. I eat the types of food I
have chosen, and the amount of food I have chosen, and then I
put down my fork, and I push myself away from the table. I
feel satisfied and full. I feel good and I appreciate how it feels
to be completely in control. Each time I eat, this image of me at
the perfect weight for me floods my mind and I feel healthy,
satisfied and full so quickly. This feeling enables me to release
all the weight I chose to.

Part 4

<u>Re-emergence</u>

This part of your self-hypnosis program is the part where you
come out of your deep relaxed state. It is important to take
some time to re-emerge because you will likely feel sleepy and
relaxed and you want to ensure you are fully wide awake
before you continue with your day. Do not skip this important
step, or you may feel groggy for a few minutes afterwards.

This self-hypnosis session has reached my subconscious mind and it feels great to change my programming to something so positive and healthy. It is time to emerge from my session with all these new ideas now part of my thinking and behaviour.

I begin to climb the staircase and I take the first step up, and I begin to feel more awake and energized, I take another step and I feel more energized and awake, with each step I take I am more ready to get back to my day.

Now as I climb the stairs I begin to emerge and energize. Now step numbers 8, 7 and 6. I continue up the stairs, 5, 4, 3, more and more energized, and I am almost ready to open my eyes. 2 and 1 and I am now all the way up the staircase, and I am ready to get back to my day, and I feel ready to enjoy being in control. I open my eyes now knowing I have had a great session which has helped me so much.

After you have completed your session

When you reach the end of your self-hypnosis session and you have opened your eyes, take a moment to ensure you are wide awake. You may wish to stretch or move around for a few minutes to make sure you are fully awake and ready to resume your activities.

Creating your own self-hypnosis script

Emily's script is based upon the specific negative programming she needed to overcome in order to release her weight. You likely have some of the same negative beliefs, so you may want to use some of the script you see above. However, it is important to think about your own negative programming. Use the "Negative Programming Worksheet" at the back of the book to create your own script, which you will use when you use your cell phone or other device to record your own self-hypnosis program.

Chapter 3

How Does Complaining Have a Negative Influence on You?

Many people overlook how damaging their complaining is to their ability to be successful. Think about it this way, when you complain you are in fact compounding the negative and focusing on how bad your situation is. Your own complaining makes you feel worse about the things that are challenging in your life and helps, in fact make these things harder to overcome.

For example, if you have a financial situation which you are finding difficult to change, you may notice you are making one or some of the following negative comments to yourself.

- Why are things so hard for me?

- Some people have all the luck.

- Some people are lucky, because they were given money.

- Rich people get all the breaks.

- The housing market is crazy.

- My parents never gave me money.

- Things are easier for other people.

- Rich people are so greedy.

These complaints become part of your own negative programming. What is true for weight loss is also true for becoming financially successful. You cannot change unless you believe you can achieve success.

Let's look at a few of these complaints and think about how they make it harder for a person to become wealthy.

My parents never gave me money

When a person makes this type of complaint, they are in fact telling themselves, that other people are responsible for their problems. If you spend your life complaining about your parents, you begin to feel sorry for yourself, and begin to feel that unless other people change, you will not be successful. The problem with this is that, chances are if your parents didn't give you money in the past, they are not likely to suddenly hand you a bunch of cash. Even though their parents are unlikely to change, many people become stuck by their complaints about them. If this type of thinking becomes ingrained in your thinking, you become stuck in the past. If your parents did not give you money, that is in the past. If you want to be successful, stop complaining about that, it is over with.

If you do notice yourself complaining about your parents, think about changing complaints about your parents into something more positive such as, "My parents did the best they could" or, "I am an adult and I make my own money."

It is important to understand that the reason your complaining should stop is because it convinces you that you cannot change, and you will find yourself unable to see any solution to your problem. Think of it this way, if you believe somebody else caused your problems, how can you see a path forward to do better for yourself? For this reason, it is essential that you stop complaining. If you do hear yourself complaining, be ready with one of your new more positive phrases such as "I am an adult and I am responsible for my own financial success."

Some people have all the luck

This is a common complaint of a person who envies somebody else's success. If you spend your time thinking about how jealous you are of what somebody else has accomplished financially, you will not have the time or energy to work on a plan to create wealth for yourself. Additionally, if your deeply held belief is that becoming wealthy is due to luck and not hard work, then there is really no motivation to even try.

It is far more likely that you will achieve better financial results when you change your belief that getting wealthy is about luck to a phrase that is more positive such as, "I plan and implement a path to my own financial success." or "I work to find new ways to create financial success each day."

Changing your thinking about your ability to succeed in this way stimulates your mind to be creative and seek a path to becoming wealthy as opposed to just sitting and feeling bad about being unlucky.

Rich people are so greedy

This complaint is one that many people have made. I cannot say whether rich people are greedy, but I do suggest that if you want to be a rich person, it makes sense to stop thinking about rich people in a negative way. The reason it is more beneficial to stop believing that the rich have negative characteristics, is that your subconscious mind will take note of this belief and if you are constantly reinforcing the negative beliefs about the rich, it will sabotage your efforts to become one of them.

Your subconscious mind would simply hear information about how terrible rich people are and that belief would likely keep you from becoming wealthy yourself. Please take time to move away from thinking negatively about the wealthy if you want to become wealthy. If you want to be wealthy think in a positive way about people with money.

Consider instead some new ways that you can think about rich people. For example, think about the efforts of people such as Bill Gates. Bill Gates, the super-rich founder of Microsoft, has more recently started a foundation which has donated millions of dollars to charity. Through his foundation he is using his money to help some of the poorest people in the world. He is using his great wealth to help others.

 Think about changing your negative beliefs about the wealthy to something more positive such as. "When I become wealthy, I will help others." Or perhaps, "Many wealthy people are making a real difference in the world." When you think of the wealthy in this new way, it creates energy in you to strive to be wealthy and do better in your own life and to also want to help those around you. If you want to be wealthy, you must think in positive ways about people who are rich.

What about complaints about weight loss and exercise?

Some typical complaints about losing weight and getting in shape include:

- Some people have it so easy because they were born with great metabolisms.
- Nobody ever helped me stay in shape.

- Why did my parents cook such fattening foods?

- Why is healthy food so bland?

- They never taught me anything about eating right in school.

- Why did I marry somebody who won't help me get healthy?

- Why won't my family help with the cooking?

These types of complaints and others become powerful programming to your subconscious mind and reinforce the idea that losing weight and getting in shape is impossible. It does not make sense to think you can keep complaining and repeatedly reinforce negative thinking and be successful in your goals to release extra weight and get in shape.

 If you want to get rid of the weight, you must stop complaining about all these things and more. If you complain in this way, you are bombarding yourself with negative programming which tells your subconscious mind that you can never overcome all the obstacles that you feel are in your way.

You may not complain yourself, but you may be listening to the complaints of others. The phrase, misery loves company, can be so true when it comes to the difficulties, we have in overcoming our bad habits. If you have friends that constantly complain about not being able to change or tell you about how they have failed to lose weight you may find yourself beginning to believe some of your negative friend's comments. Try to align yourself with friends who have a positive attitude and support you in your goal to change. Listening to negative friends could sabotage your ability to lose weight.

Of course, it doesn't mean you can't talk to your friends about your weight loss challenges but the way you discuss them makes a difference. For example, let's pretend you spent 30 minutes relaxing and doing your self-hypnosis before you left the house. You packed your healthy food for the day, and you have your running shoes in your bag because you are going to take a walk after you eat your lunch.

Imagine now, that you are sitting at your desk and your co-worker drops by to chat. Your co-worker begins to talk about how much they hate exercise and how she would rather eat chips for lunch because it helps her to relax. This scenario could be challenging for you, because you are working hard to change your own beliefs and because your own beliefs have been built up over decades and have become the programming in your subconscious mind.

The last thing you want to do is join in with these complaints as they could undermine the work you have been doing to create your own new beliefs. Perhaps you could remind your friend that you have committed yourself to making changes.

Addressing your friend's negative comments is important. Your commitment to changing your own thinking could be undermined by people who do not realize they are having a negative effect upon you. It would be beneficial to decide not to engage in this type of complaining or negativity. You must keep your own thoughts positive and aligned with your new thinking. Keep in mind your beliefs are what control your actions. This makes it very important that you never engage in complaining and refrain from joining in on conversations about how hard it is to lose weight.

There are several ways to cope with somebody else's negative comments or complaining. One way is to try to avoid certain people or excuse yourself if they are saying things that are negative. You could also tell them you are changing your own thinking and ask them to be supportive. Thirdly, it would be beneficial for the co-worker or friend to join you in your efforts to eat better or get more exercise. Perhaps they could join you on a walk.

Maybe asking people to have a more positive attitude may seem a bit weird at first and that is ok. Keep in mind that your old ways of doing things did not work that well for you. Positive attitudes and comments add to your subconscious programming and because our goal here is to make changes to that level of your thinking, keeping the negative comments of others to a minimum, is important.

You may also have people in your life that could be described as "enablers". These people would be anybody who might want you to in some small way to fail. For example, you may have a friend that you have been in the habit of getting together to eat cheesecake with every Friday night.

 You may worry that your friend will feel left behind or upset to hear that you won't be having your usual cheesecake date. Despite this person being a friend, they might want to undermine you because they want you to continue to meet with them each week. Your friendship and your weekly date may be something they look very forward each week and they may not want things to change. Their disappointment in you could be upsetting to you and if your friend is important to you, you may feel pressure to give up on your own goals just to avoid upsetting a good friend.

Enablers have their own reasons for wanting you to keep doing the things you have always done. Perhaps, they enjoy things as they are, and are comfortable with carrying some extra weight. Perhaps, they love cooking for friends and family, and may feel like you don't love them as much if you change your mind about wanting to eat less.

Parents can sometimes be enablers. Your parents may have a long history of enabling your poor habits. For example, family gatherings may be always done at the same household in the same way. Perhaps Sunday afternoons have always been about watching the big game with your father. The big game may involve the same types of snacks you have been eating for years. Be aware that these types of scenarios are common, but like other enablers, parents can inadvertently undermine your progress.

Perhaps your friend would be fine with changing your weekly cheesecake date to a coffee and a walk. Chances are one of the main reasons you get together is so you can enjoy some social time. In any case, choosing how you would like to handle this situation before it becomes something that keeps you from being successful is important. Once you have chosen how this situation will be handled, then make it part of your script.

Always keep in mind that you will be more successful when you associate yourself with positive supportive people, so do all you can to make friends and family part of your support system.

If parents or others insist on you continuing to behave the way you always have even though they know you want to improve your life, it may be a good idea to speak to them about what your goals are and what you have been doing to change. You may also ask them to join in with what you are doing, or to change some of the things they have been doing.

Parents, husbands, and kids can change. Friends can learn about new ways to eat and socialize. Perhaps everybody would enjoy trying some new foods, or some new activities.

It is extremely beneficial that you think about what the pitfalls may be and decide the best way to handle your social interactions with your family and friends. It is important that you include how you will handle these situations in your self-hypnosis script. For example, you may include suggestions such as the following.

I enjoy my weekly cheesecake date with my friend, and we have our cheesecake and then go for a walk. We walk for 30 minutes and we both benefit from our physical exercise, and we enjoy our social time more than ever.

I enjoy a snack with my father during the game, and I have one small bowl and feel satisfied. Our time together continues to be important to me and I enjoy our time more and more.

I enjoy the meals my mother cooks, and I have one portion and then leave the table feeling very satisfied. I go for a thirty-minute walk afterwards and my family joins me and we all enjoy the time we have together in nature. Our children benefit too, because we all spend more time together talking and engaging in healthy activities.

Deciding ahead of time how you will handle some of the difficulties you know will come up, is a great way to avoid any surprises. If you are prepared and ready for challenges, then you will find you can continue to be successful. If you do not plan for each of these situations, you will not know how to handle them and may eat more than you intended to and then perhaps feel you have failed.
Nobody is saying you cannot enjoy special occasions or events. But, if you have decided how you will handle them, and then add it to your script you will continue to be in control and be successful. Keep in mind your goal is to create

new programming which creates new beliefs and new

habits.

Think for a moment about a client who may enjoy the Sunday afternoon game with their father. If he or she decided they would continue to enjoy watching the game with him, and they have decided that they will have one small bowl of a snack they enjoy, and they have prepared to handle this situation in this manner they will be successful.

The benefit of experiencing successes like the one described above is that it builds upon the subconscious programming you have already been working to establish. When you experience success, that great feeling becomes part of your new programming.

Understanding your own programming

When it comes to you and your success, it is important to understand your own beliefs and how they are keeping you from doing what you really want to do. Your own negative programming could be beliefs that you have been carrying around for years, or quite likely, decades. The following negative beliefs could be the reason you have been unable to get in shape and lose weight.

Review the following chart of negative beliefs and see if any of these beliefs sound familiar to you. The reasons may be why you have been unable to release the weight you want to lose.

Common negative beliefs that keep people from losing weight

I have always been overweight.
I love junk food too much to give it up.
Dieting is too hard.
People always gain the weight back.
I am too lazy.
It is easier to be overweight.
I am happy being overweight.
People like me the way I am.
My family will be upset if I lose weight.
I don't know what to do.
I would rather lay on the couch.
I hate exercise.

You likely have other beliefs about weight loss, add them to the list above. The list above is not every reason that people can't lose weight or get in shape, but it is a good starting point. If you have said or thought any of the phrases from the above list, to yourself once, there is a good chance you have said it to yourself repeatedly. It is likely that you have said these things to yourself thousands of times.

Imagine the impact saying these types of things to yourself repeatedly over the course of several years, or even decades. It is unlikely that you will be successful in losing weight or getting into shape if your underlying beliefs keep telling you will fail. That is why changing these beliefs at the sub-conscious level is so important.

These beliefs block us from achieving what we want and keep us from changing. Imagine the impact of saying these types of things to yourself repeatedly over the course of several years, or even decades. It is unlikely that you will be successful in losing weight if your underlying beliefs tell you that you will fail. That is why changing these beliefs at the subconscious level is so important.

Think about the pregnant smoker

An interesting example of how programming can be changed quickly at the subconscious level, is the example of a woman who quits smoking as soon as she gets the good news that she will soon be a mother. The reason this woman can switch from being a smoker to a non-smoker so easily is because the news of motherhood creates new programming that overrides the old programming instantly. She may have had thoughts such as "I can't change, I like smoking too much, I have always been a smoker, all my friends are smokers" as well as, "smoking is very important to me."

While these beliefs may have had her stuck as a lifetime smoker before her pregnancy, these thoughts become overwritten instantaneously, in much the same way new programming changes the way a computer operates.

Her new beliefs could include the following health issues that a doctor would likely share with a mother-to-be who is a smoker.

- Smoking can cause low birth weights

- Smoking could cause my baby to have asthma

- Smoking robs my baby of oxygen

- Mothers-to-be should not smoke

These medical facts would be taken seriously by the mother-to-be and cause instant changes to the programming in the subconscious mind. These new beliefs become the new programming that makes quitting smoking easy for this new mother.

The subconscious mind can be programmed

In order to reprogram the subconscious mind, the negative programming must be rewritten with new programming. We know that negative beliefs at the subconscious level led to negative outcomes. The opposite is also true. New positive programming will give new and positive outcomes. In order to create new thoughts and beliefs one must reach the subconscious mind through the techniques of self-hypnosis.

Chapter 4

Preparing For Successful Self-Hypnosis

Hypnosis is something we may think we know about from countless television shows and movies. In these programs hypnosis is seen as something spooky sometimes associated with mad scientists. Do not worry about these negative images. We are simply talking about learning how to eliminate our negative beliefs and replacing them with positive programming.

When we talk about self-hypnosis, we are learning to induce a deeply relaxed state in order to allow the subconscious mind to be reached for the purpose of changing the programming there. The sleepy dreamlike state is important for reaching the subconscious mind.

When you are working with a Hypnotherapist, they will use a variety of techniques to ensure you reach a deeply relaxed state. When you are doing self-hypnosis, you will be responsible for reaching the state on your own. There are several scripts that can be found at the end of this book that will enable you to reach the state you need to reach to have a successful self-hypnosis session.

Choose the one that works best for you and record it on your cellphone or any other recording device, so you can listen to it along with your suggestions, post-hypnotic suggestions and suggestions to re-emerge.

You may be wondering if self-hypnosis is effective. The answer is yes, many people have had excellent results in making the changes they crave. Self-hypnosis can be just as effective as working with a hypnotherapist provided you take time when you read this book to ensure you understand how each part works.

It may be a good idea for some people to experiment with just doing the induction (reaching the deeply relaxed state). It is important that your mind and body are completely relaxed because in this state the subconscious mind is open to suggestions. This is the state that works best for self-hypnosis.

The hypnotic state is sleep-like in some ways, but it is also quite different. While we are sleeping, we are not aware of what is happening around us, even though the mind is active. While we are asleep, we cannot accept the suggestions given to the subconscious mind. We instead need to be relaxed, but awake.

If you find you are falling asleep, try sitting up slightly instead of laying down. You could perhaps try another time of day. Experiment to find out what works best for you. Hypnosis cannot help you if you are asleep.

It is also important that you take time to determine what your negative programming consists of. I suggest using a journal and writing down any negative thoughts regarding your goal, that enter your mind. If you do this for three or more days you will notice patterns in your thoughts, and it will help you become aware of what you need to work on.

When you have a list that you are satisfied with, create new positive programming that will replace these negative thoughts. These new positive suggestions will form the basis of your self-hypnosis script that you will record on your phone. Suggestion directly follow your induction. There are examples at the end of the book that show you how to turn negative programming into positive suggestions.

.

You may find it helpful to think about what kind of eating program you want to follow. You could check out the library or do some research online. Find something that is reasonable that does not require a drastic reduction in calories. Your goal is to find a sensible and reasonable way to eat. This means something like an all-grapefruit diet is not what you are looking for.

Choose an eating plan that is moderate and something you could do long-term. Depending on your budget you could also speak to a nutritionist. Another option is to investigate some of the companies that deliver a box of ingredients each week, with recipe cards so you can cook healthy food without having to shop.

Decide about what type of exercise will be best for you. This is a conversation that you should have with your doctor, who may have suggestions as to what is most appropriate for you.

After speaking to your doctor decide what type of exercise is going to work with your schedule, and budget. If you like aerobic classes or dance classes these would be good options for you. It is important that you choose something you enjoy which makes it so much easier to be successful.

If you think walking would be the exercise for you, choose a time that is convenient and a place that is easily accessible. Buy a new set of shoes if you need to, and perhaps ask a friend or relative to join you.

It is always easier to be successful if you spend some time to think about the easiest way to be successful, prepare to be successful, and add your plans to your self-hypnosis script.

It is also a good idea to keep in mind that as time goes on, you may find it necessary to change your self-hypnosis program.

For example, you may be going on a vacation, and you may want to handle things differently. That is ok. Simply think about what your goals will be while you are away and adjust your script. You have the power to make changes quite easily. The secret is to take a bit of time to think about your goal and adjust accordingly.

.

Chapter 5

Cheryl's Story

Let's talk about techniques which will enable you to reach the subconscious mind, which will allow you to change the negative programming that is found there.

Review the list of negative beliefs found in chapter 3. This list includes common negative programming that prevents people from losing weight and getting fit. Take some time to review it and think about the beliefs you have about your own goals to lose weight, get healthy and get in shape. Check off the ones that you know are part of your programming. Then, add any other ones that have been part of your programming, and which have been keeping you stuck. Take your time with this list, as it is important to try to work on these beliefs all at once.

<u>Please keep in mind that:</u>

New programming that comes from our experiences can do one of two things:

Negative Thoughts, Ideas and Experiences → They reinforce negative beliefs that are already there. They add power to those negative beliefs, they make them more powerful.

Positive Thoughts, Ideas and Experiences → They have the power to rewrite or override the negative ones and with time and repetition can cause changes to core programming which changes our beliefs and our behaviours.

After you have begun working to reprogram your subconscious mind, you may discover that you have other programming that also needs to be addressed. Add any other beliefs that come up as you discover them. It is important to be aware of as many of these beliefs as possible. These beliefs are keeping you from reaching your goal and they need to be addressed. Please keep in mind that we are complex beings and there may be several negative beliefs that have accumulated over the years.

Some people feel a deep sense of sadness when they read their list of negative programming. Our negative beliefs often have a great deal of emotion attached to them. Emotions that come up when we begin to think about our programming may include, shame, embarrassment, anger or sadness. This emotional component is what makes our programming so powerful. If you experience these types of emotions when you begin to work on your list of negative self-talk, it is completely normal.

You may wish to spend time working on understanding the root of these emotions, and perhaps add to the script you will be making in order to feel more comfortable with the emotions related to your weight. This is not something that comes up for everybody when they begin to think about their beliefs. However, you may realize you have a great deal of "baggage" that you have been carrying around. As you learn more about your negative programming, simply add any new beliefs to the list as they come up. You will use the items on your list to create suggestions for yourself.

You must decide to overcome these beliefs which have been programming your behaviour. Remember, without making a change to your beliefs you cannot change your behaviour. Remember too, if your underlying programming says, "I can never lose weight", there is no way you can be successful.

Keep in mind, if you carry these beliefs at the subconscious level, it is probable that you have repeated the same thoughts over and over again. That is what makes them powerful. That is why, reading your list and making a commitment to make a change is so important.

In my work with clients who are overweight I have often worked with clients who are holding on to a great deal of shame related to their body and their weight. I worked with one such woman, named Cheryl who told a story about being heavy as a child. She described being teased by other kids, and feelings of embarrassment about her body.

Cheryl's story

In our initial conversation, Cheryl described her early life. Her mother was overweight, and she and her mother visited Doctor's offices, and began weight loss programs together. Many of her family members such as aunts and her grandmother were also heavy and while attending these appointments and programs, a narrative about the family's difficulties in losing weight became a part of Cheryl's programming. There were feelings of hopelessness and the belief that nobody in the family had ever been successful which made Cheryl think it was pointless to even try.

The appointments with Doctor's and the trips to weight loss groups made Cheryl feel like she had a problem that none of her friends at school faced. She would sometimes take salads and what she called "diet food" in her lunches which caused a lot of embarrassment and teasing. Other times when she and her mom would go off their diets, she would have sweets and all kinds of fattening foods in her lunch. Kids began to realize that she had failed in her attempt to lose weight and called her all kinds of upsetting names.

Despite being a child Cheryl felt a great deal of shame about her body and began to hate any kind of physical activity because she knew it would be difficult and that kids would laugh at her. Her mom would sometimes write her a note so that she could get out of gym class because Cheryl could become quite distraught at times.

She faced criticism about her eating habits at home as well. Her parents would criticize her if she put too much food on her plate and if she wanted to have any kind of snack. She felt she was always disappointing them and her shame about wanting snacks lead her to sometimes sneak food into her bedroom and eat it hurriedly late at night. She always felt fearful that she would be caught with snacks in her room, and as such she ate very quickly so nobody would find out her secret.

These practices caused a great deal of embarrassment and Cheryl had to be coaxed to reveal that she had been sneaking food when she was a child. Cheryl still felt even as an adult that her family was watching her. She even felt like her friends and co-workers judged her every time put something in her mouth.

Cheryl was close to tears when she talked about how difficult it had been to grow up being overweight. She was teased when she ate healthy food, and ridiculed when she ate so called "fattening" food. She began to battle with her mom about dieting and her weight, which Cheryl to have a great deal of resentment and anger towards her mother.

Cheryl eventually resigned herself to the idea that she would be overweight for the rest of her life and was very conflicted about whether she should even try to get her weight and health under control. Trying hypnosis was a last-ditch attempt and Cheryl told me she had little hope that hypnosis could turn things around for her.

Cheryl contacted me initially because several family members were beginning to have health concerns such as diabetes, heart related illnesses, and joint problems. Cheryl was becoming scared that if she did not do something about her own weight, that she too would face health concerns as she got older. She was desperate to take off the weight she had been carrying and did not feel very hopeful that she could do something she had been told was so difficult.

I convinced Cheryl to spend time thinking about her own programming and to talk about it with her family. She began to understand that her beliefs had been programmed early in her life and that they were holding her back from making changes. She also realized that she could not change her weight until she overcame her negative beliefs. I reminded Cheryl that negative programming will always be stronger than willpower.

Cheryl's feelings about losing weight included a lot of negative emotional programming which is shared in the chart below. This is typical, especially if a person has been overweight since childhood.

Negative emotions which began in our childhoods often hold us back as adults. I explained to Cheryl how these deeply held beliefs become our programming and this programming in our subconscious mind is what shapes our lives and makes us who we are.

I expressed to Cheryl that if she held onto the beliefs she had learned early in her life she could never lose weight. After speaking to Cheryl and learning more about her childhood, I created a script that she could use in order to reduce her weight. I then taught her how to reach a deep state of relaxation so she could reach her subconscious mind in order to change the negative programming to positive programming.

Cheryl was initially skeptical but once she began listening to her self-hypnosis script she felt hope for the first time in decades, and she was very successful in reducing her weight. She realized that she had been held back by the beliefs she held.

She was not initially aware that these powerful beliefs had been the source of her difficulties. Once Cheryl began to understand her beliefs and began working on changing them, the weight she had been holding onto began to disappear. Cheryl eventually lost all the weight she wanted to and uses her script to help keep her at a comfortable weight.

Cheryl's list of negative programming included the following beliefs

My family has always been overweight.
When my family members lose weight, they always gain it back.
My family loves socializing which always means overeating.
Gyms are for athletic people who know how to exercise.
People at the gym will laugh at me.
My family will be upset if I lose weight.
Losing weight is too hard.

Cheryl's self-hypnosis script

To follow is the self-hypnosis script Cheryl used to reduce her weight and keep it from returning. The script was based upon the assessment she completed which helped determine what programming in her subconscious mind needed to be addressed.

Cheryl initially listened to her self-hypnosis recording twice per day but two months, she noticed she felt so good, and so strong, that she just needed to listen to it once per day. Once she had reduced her weight to where she wanted it to be, she listened to it less frequently as she had internalized all the new programming and had proved to herself that she could be successful and did not have to have the same weight loss story that her parents and family had.

Cheryl typically laid back in comfortable chair and listened through headphones to the script she had recorded on her phone.

Deep relaxation/induction

With my eyes closed, I imagine myself in front of an elevator. This elevator is special, and when I get into it, it takes me deep down into a very relaxed state, and as the elevator takes me down, each floor takes me to a deeper place of relaxation.

I see the doors open and I walk onto the elevator, I am alone, and I feel comfortable, safe and calm. The doors close silently. I notice the keypad and there is only one button, and I calmly reach out and press it. The elevator begins to descend silently. I notice that the elevator is slowly descending and as it slowly moves downward, I find myself relaxing more and more. The elevator gently descends lower and lower and I gently relax. Each floor that we pass takes me deeper, and I notice my body relaxes more and more.

I love the feeling of relaxation, so I allow myself to become more and more relaxed. The elevator silently goes deeper and so do I.

I am now halfway to full and complete relaxation now, and I want to go deeper, so, as the elevator descends so do I. Each part of me gently relaxing and gently feeling more calm, more and more peaceful, and more and more relaxed. I feel myself breathe in and exhale deeply and now I am more and more relaxed.

One more deep inhale and exhale and now almost completely relaxed. Now another deep breath and I allow myself to be fully relaxed, deeply relaxed now, calm, and peaceful. I am feeling good and feeing fully relaxed and ready to take in all the new information that changes my body mind and spirit.

The elevator doors open now, and I look out and notice a picture hanging on the wall. It is a picture of me at the perfect weight for me. I look at the picture and I realize that it is me looking happy and confident. I walk over towards the picture, and I take some time now to look at myself, from head to toe. I notice my face and my neck, my body, my arms and legs. I notice every part of me at the perfect weight. I look healthy, slim, strong, energetic and I know I am reaching the perfect weight for me.

Suggestions

I love my family, and they love me. They have faced challenges with their weight, and that is their story. I am very different from them. I have a mind of my own. My life is my own and creating changes in my life is a normal part of growing up. Reaching my perfect weight is about changing my habits. Their habits belong to them, and I choose to create my own programming which creates new beliefs, new feelings and new habits for me.

I am ready to change and I am choosing now to create a new story for myself. I can reduce the weight I no longer want. Change is a perfectly natural part of life; people change all of the time and now I am changing. People change jobs, change homes and change is normal and now I am changing my weight. The change to my programming means I remove the weight from my body, and I keep it off for good. I know the weight stays off because I have changed my programming in my subconscious mind. I relax knowing the programming changes, the beliefs change, and the weight comes off my body and it stays off permanently. It is perfectly natural to change, and it is perfectly natural for the weight to leave my body.

I took time to find an eating plan that works for me. I read, I talked to friends, and now I know what to eat, and how to eat. I have found a good plan that I know works for me. I chose a plan, and it is successful, and I am successful, and I reduce my weight in a natural easy way.

I love my family and we continue to socialize. We have fun doing all the fun things we have always done. I enjoy our time together. I have chosen a new way to live my life and now when I socialize with them, I simply eat a little differently than I used to. If they notice, I explain I am eating a little differently so I can keep my heart healthy and keep my joints healthy. I expect them to be supportive and helpful. I expect them to be kind. If that is not the case, I am good. It is important to me to take the weight off my body. I continue to do well, and the weight leaves my body. I am strong and I am eating a little differently and that is great.

I am enjoying my exercise program. I now know how much I enjoy riding a bike. The breeze, the beauty of nature. I can go for ten minutes or an hour, it depends on how I feel. I ride my bike four or more times a week. It is surprising how much I enjoy being on my bike, I feel good, and I notice how strong my legs feel and I notice now when I walk up a flight of stairs it seems so much easier.

My bike is so fun, and it brings me health and peace. It helps me let the weight go and I feel so good. When the weather cools down, I go for a walk around my neighbourhood and I enjoy it so much. I breathe deeply and enjoy the fresh air and the great feeling I have in my body. Walking helps my body, my mind and my spirit. I walk and I reduce my weight.

Post-hypnotic suggestions

Each time before I eat, be it a snack or a meal, the image of me at the perfect weight I have chosen for myself, floods my mind. Just before I take in food, I see how good my body looks and feels at the perfect weight for me. I notice my face looks healthy, my eyes are bright, and I have a relaxed peaceful look on my face. This image makes me feel strong, and motivated.

I also notice my arms are strong and slim, my chest and back are the right shape and size and these parts of body look great in the clothing I wear. My waist is trim and fit perfectly into the clothing I choose.

My legs are strong, and my jeans and workout clothing feel good and look good. I enjoy wearing my clothing. I enjoy choosing clothing that looks good and feels good. My figure is attractive, and I feel healthy strong and attractive. The thought of my body at the perfect weight for me floods my mind each time I eat. It motivates me and makes me successful.

Re-emergence

My self-hypnosis session was excellent today. The suggestions I gave myself make me a success. I am ready to re-emerge and feel wide awake and energetic. I imagine I am back in front of the elevator door, and it is time to go back up and get back to my day.

I walk calmly into the elevator. There is one button which has an up arrow. I am ten floors down and I press the button and the elevator begins to slowly and silently move upward. I am moving upwards and emerging, I move upward, and I am beginning to feel more energetic, I am beginning to feel more awake. The elevator continues to move upward, and I am feeling more and more awake, more and more lively. The elevator is halfway to the surface, and I gently move my limbs as I continue upward to the surface, each floor taking me towards the surface. I am almost there now, and I move my body a little bit more and I begin to feel lively and awake.

I am at the surface now and I feel good, lively, healthy and awake and ready for my day. The elevator doors open, and I am at the surface. I feel good, I feel hopeful and healthy,

Energetic now, lively and awake, awake, awake and I am ready for my day, feeling so good. I am ready to open my eyes.

I open my eyes.

After you re-emerge

When you re-emerge take a moment to open your eyes, stretch for a few moments, take some deep breaths to ensure you are wide awake. When you have done so and are fully aware, you can return to your day.

Cheryl was a very successful client, and her success helped her mother reduce her weight as well. Her mother was extremely happy for Cheryl when she began to slim down. Cheryl's mother did not initially think that self-hypnosis would work for her and had a negative attitude towards trying it for herself.

However, after a few months of observing Cheryl and listening to what Cheryl said about what had been helping her, her mother began to be interested in what it was that was helping Cheryl to be so successful. Cheryl helped her mom complete the self-assessment and helped her record her own personalized weight reduction script.

Her mother also had very good results. She lost a great deal of the weight that she had been holding onto for decades. The greatest benefit to Cheryl's mother was the improvements to her health. Her high blood pressure was normal for the first time in many years. Her joint problems virtually disappeared as well. The two women also improved their relationship with one another and became closer as a result of the new understanding they had about themselves and each other.

Chapter 6

Sarah's Story

Sarah is a mother of two kids, a 7-year-old and a 5-year-old. She had led a healthy active lifestyle and was happy with her body weight up until the birth of her children. She gained 40 pounds during the pregnancy of her first child. She lost most of the weight after her first child was born. She gained 40 pounds with her second child as well. This weight was far more difficult to release, and she found that she had no time or energy to spend on taking the weight off with two children to take care of.

By the time I met her she was 50 pounds overweight, exhausted and she was feeling demoralized. She described how her life felt out of control and it was easy to see how she had become overwhelmed when she thought about trying to reduce her weight.

Sarah's husband worked out of town a great deal, which meant she had to take care of the children on her own most of the time. Prior to the birth of her first child Sarah and her husband had moved and she had very little family close by. She had yet to establish any new friendships. She loved her children, but they were extremely active, and she went to bed each night feeling exhausted.

Sarah knew she wanted to make some changes to her life, including getting her weight under control so she could feel more energetic, and healthy. She was fearful that she could become depressed if she did not do something about the feeling of being stuck. She contacted me because she was confused about what to do in order to feel better and get back to the way she felt about herself just a few short years before.

Sarah's negative beliefs about her weight and getting in shape

I am too busy to deal with my weight right now.
Looking attractive is not important now that I am married.
It is selfish to take time away from my kids to go to the gym.
I am too busy to prepare healthy food.
I can lose weight later when the kids are older.
Moms are often overweight.
A lot of women can't lose weight after having kids.
Once the kids are older, I can focus on this stuff.
I can't lose weight until I have help from my husband.
I can't find new friends until I look better.
It is terrible to try to focus on my weight when I am a mother.
I will have to cook separate meals for my kids and husband.

After Sarah had spent some time putting together her list, she began to understand that some of the beliefs that she had accumulated since the birth of the kids were harming her. She also realized that there were some things that she could do without help from her husband, and there were also some things that she could discuss with him so that they could work on things together.

Sarah had never spoken to husband very much about how she was feeling. He knew of course that she had gained weight and he had never said anything negative about it. He was a supportive husband, but he too, had gained weight since they had married, and the poor eating habits and sedentary lifestyle were issues for him as well.

Sarah realized that the couple should talk about the issue of how they were living their lives together for her to be successful.

After our initial discussion about Sarah's life, she began to see how her beliefs were responsible for her inability to take off the weight she wanted to lose. She and I worked together to create a script which she would use to overcome the programming in her subconscious mind which had accumulated there since the birth of her children.

We also realized that some of the programming had been there for longer and she reflected upon how she had listened to her mother and aunts discuss weight and childbirth on numerous occasions and that what she heard them say had always been a part of her belief system. However, this part of her programming had never concerned her until she too had children. Once she was a mother these long-held myths became stumbling blocks for her. She understood these beliefs were powerful, and that no progress could be made without changes to her subconscious programming.

 Like my client Cheryl, Sarah had heard a variety of myths about weight loss from other women in her family. Sarah realized that the things she heard as a girl had become stuck in her mind and were strong and powerful. Our parents of course do not try to sabotage us, but when children overhear parents repeating the same stories and complaints over and over again, the beliefs become powerful.

When I asked Sarah about certain beliefs such as: It is selfish to take time for yourself to go to the gym or prepare healthy foods, she told me about listening to her mother talk to her friends about their own challenges with their weight.

She recalled hearing comments like these from the time she was a young girl, meaning that she had held onto the programming for decades without realizing that listening to these older women had shaped her beliefs about weight and motherhood. They had also been responsible for her own beliefs about weight and motherhood.

Before Sarah had become pregnant, she had never really thought about her weight or what she ate. I questioned her about that, and she told me that when she was young, she had often heard that the women she knew, only had difficulty with their weight after the birth of their children. We understood that we had to overcome beliefs around this topic in order for Sarah to take off the weight.

Sarah and I discussed these beliefs and how important it is to address negative programming. Together we created some new positive programming, which became the basis for her self-hypnosis script.

Sarah's New Positive Programming

Moms are often fit and in shape.
Being a great mom is easier when I am in shape.
I am happier around my family when I get exercise.
I have more energy when I take some time for myself.
I am a calm and happy mom when I feel fit.
The whole family benefits from healthy food.
I have three hours a week to get to a yoga class.
It is a good idea to set healthy examples for my kids.

I asked her to commit to a routine of self-hypnosis so that she could in a sense "reset" her ideas about her weight and fitness so she could be more like she was before the birth of her children.

Sarah was also feeling overwhelmed by all the information

available about diets and healthy eating. When she first got married, she and her husband had been very active, and Sarah never really thought about what she should be eating, and her weight was never an issue.

She started by reading a few books about different eating plans, but nothing really interested her. She decided that she would need the assistance of a nutritionist, to help her create a good plan for her, and help her ensure her kids were also eating healthier. She also asked her husband to join her at the nutritionist so that eating in a healthier way was something they worked on together as opposed to it being something that she was forcing onto him.

Her husband was supportive of Sarah's decision to enlist a professional to help create a plan for the whole family. He understood that Sarah's weight was making her unhappy and he agreed that the whole family could benefit from eating healthier food and he himself remembered how much better he felt when he was at a more comfortable weight.

One important thing to keep in mind is that Sarah's issues with her weight only began when she had a change in her circumstances. She may have never had an issue with her weight had she not become a mother. This is certainly not unusual, especially for women who have listened in on conversations from older female relatives.

Sara and I discussed how things had changed for her. Prior to the birth of her kids, Sarah believed the following about her ability to stay in shape and maintain her weight.

Sarah's Beliefs About Her Weight, Before the Birth of Her Children

I enjoy exercise.
My social life involves physical activity.
Exercise makes life easier.
Exercise helps me cope with life.
Being active reduces my stress.
I feel good about my weight.
I like the way my body looks.
I like the way I look in my clothes.
It is easy to maintain my weight.
Eating junk food makes me feel sluggish.
I enjoy eating healthy food.
I hate when my clothes feel tight.
I can maintain my weight by hiking and enjoying the outdoors.

Sarah's self-hypnosis script

Sarah was excited about getting started with self-hypnosis. She had previous experience with yoga and meditation, and she knew she would have no trouble with reaching a relaxed state. She chose to do what is called a progressive type of relaxation for her self-hypnosis sessions which she knew would work well for her. A progressive type of script simply means she would relax one body part at a time until her whole body was fully relaxed.

Sarah found she was too busy to do her script right away in the morning, so she woke up and got her kids ready for school, and then once the house was quiet, she would take time to get comfortable and do her self-hypnosis script then. She found this worked well in another way as well. Sarah did not like to wear headphones so when the house was empty, she could play her script which she had recorded on her phone without having to put on headphones.

Induction/relaxation

I am taking the time now to relax and do something great for myself. I relax myself and I feel so good. I take a moment to get nice and comfortable. I make sure the temperature is right for me, I make sure I am laying back in a comfortable position which feels so good.

The first thing I do is tighten every part of my body. I make tight fists; I lift my legs and tighten all the muscles in my feet and legs. I do the same with my arms and hands. I scrunch up my face and my eyes. I take a deep breath and let my whole body relax at once, and as it relaxes, I let it sink down more and more relaxed and each part of my body feels so good.

I think about my feet and legs, and I let all the muscles relax even more, all the muscles go soft and relaxed, and it feels so good. I think about my lower back and my stomach and chest and let those areas go smooth and soft and so relaxed and it feels so good. I check in and make sure my chest feels relaxed, if I am holding anything there or my breath isn't smooth, I relax it completely, I let it go and it feels so good.

I turn my attention to my neck and my head, and I allow the muscles in my neck and face to relax, go loose and limp and relaxed. It feels good to relax and let go completely and I take a moment now, I scan my body, and any area that is not fully relaxed, I relax now. My breath is even, I feel calm and peaceful.

It feels so good, and I am ready for all the beneficial suggestions to reach my sub-conscious mind.

Suggestions

I am in very relaxed state so that the suggestions that I give my subconscious mind have a powerful effect on me. I have chosen to release extra weight now. My decision is good for me and good for my family. It is easier to be a great mom when I am taking good care of myself. I like the boost of energy I get from eating healthy food, I like the energy I have, and my kids benefit from my energy. I find doing all the activities I enjoy doing with my kids are so much easier. My kids benefit from my energy, and I feel calmer, and when I am feeling great, being a mom just works better.

One thing I really enjoy doing is taking time to do yoga after the kids go to school each day. I remember how I felt when I did yoga before the kids came along. My muscles were firm and strong, I reflect on each part of my body, and I am aware that when I did yoga regularly my body felt great.

I love that feeling, and yoga benefits me and benefits my whole family.

Yoga takes me four hours per week, and I have decided to go to the yoga studio near my house. I walk there and do the 9:30 class four mornings each week. I drop off my kids at the bus stop, and that gives me time to do my self-hypnosis session and then walk for ten minutes until I reach the yoga studio.

 I know how great this routine is for me. The fresh air, the time in nature, and time out of the house is something that I really enjoy and so I look forward to this bit of time I give myself.

Starting my new yoga routine is a benefit to me. I get stronger, I release weight, my mind is clear, I feel healthy, I feel energetic and I feel confident. My family benefits as much as I do. Doing yoga calms me and that benefits my family as well.

Doing yoga helps me sleep better at night and that benefits my family. Doing yoga makes me stronger and that benefits my family. Yoga is a benefit to me and my family. We all benefit from my new routine.

I enjoy being part of a community. I meet new people at the yoga class. Many of the people who go there are women who are stay at home moms and we have a lot in common. I get to know them as we take classes at the same time each day. This is where my new friendships grow. I also realize having friends in my new city is important. I look for mom and kid programs in my community, I look for opportunities to volunteer at school and I grow my network of friends there as well. I take my kids out to the park after school for fresh air and exercise.

I begin to see the same people at the park and new opportunities, for friendships grow. Having friends is important to me. My new city is filled with families with kids, and I seek opportunities to meet new friends and my circle of friends grows quickly.

Now that I have decided that I eat healthier food, I feel so much better. I feel great about the plan my nutritionist made for me. She made a great plan for me based upon the needs of my body. We developed some great plans, and I am excited about the new recipes I am trying. I also have a great plan for my kids. Their lunches and snacks are more nutritious, and they continue to enjoy the foods I choose for them.

I realize the changes I have decided to make are great for the entire family. My husband is so supportive, and it was great to hear he is ready to eat better as well. We have made some great decisions together and we all benefit. He has begun to plan and shop for meals when he is home on the weekends. This gives me a break, and he has begun to have the kids cook with him, giving them all valuable time together.

I enjoy the new healthy way I am eating. I feel so good and so energized. I feel strong and powerful, and my body looks great and feels great as I release the weight I have been carrying.

My kids enjoy the new foods, which makes mealtimes easy. I have discovered recipes that are nutritious and which my kids also enjoy. We all eat better and the time I took to make better choices for myself and for my family, has turned out to be a great benefit for all of us. Day by day and week by week the whole family is healthier. We look and feel stronger and stronger. I know the decisions I have made benefit my entire family.

Post-hypnotic suggestions

I know how great I look at the perfect weight for me. Each time I eat a meal or a snack, the image of myself at the perfect weight for me fills my mind and energizes me to continue with all the changes I have made. I take a moment to see that image clearly in my mind. I see my face, slim and healthy, bright, and healthy. I see my neck and my chest and my arms. They look strong and fit, and they look great at the perfect size and shape for me.

I also see in my mind, my stomach and waist. They look trim and my clothing fits so well. My jeans look great, they are comfortable, and I feel great when I put them on. When I am dressing up and when I am wearing summer clothing like dresses, shorts and workout gear, I look great.

My legs look fit and strong. I like the size of them and the shape of them and they look great when I am wearing jeans, and when I am dressing up and when I am wearing summer clothing like dresses, shorts and workout gear.

I look great, and each time I eat, the image of me at the perfect weight for me, floods into my mind. I see myself in my mind and I feel strong and motivated, and I am loving that feeling of control and energy. Each time I eat a meal or snack, the image of myself at the perfect weight for me floods my mind. When I eat the meal or snack, I have planned for myself I feel very satisfied and strong.

Re-emergence

I have had a great self-hypnosis session and it is time to re-emerge and to go on to have a great day, a successful day. The suggestions I have given myself are now part of my programing and the changes to my subconscious mind guide my new thoughts, beliefs and actions.

I count from 10 to one in a moment and as I do I re-emerge to being fully alert and awake, wide, wide awake.

10   I begin to emerge slowly coming wide awake.

9   More awake now feeling myself begin to feel more alert and ready for my day.

8   More awake feeling good, feeling more alert and feeling more awake.

7   More alert now more awake, ready for a great day.

6   Feeling good 10 times more alert now, 10 times more awake.

5   Halfway there now and feeling lively.

4   Almost ready now, almost fully emerged.

3   Feeling lively, alert emerging and full of energy.

2   Feeling good, feeling awake, almost ready for my day.

1   Fully alert now, I open my eyes, and I raise my hands
        and shake them, I move my head gently.

Alert and ready for my day. I stand up, stretch my body, I feel good, I feel alert, I am ready for a great day, ready for a successful day.

Sarah began to lose weight soon after she began to use self-hypnosis to change her programming. She found a way to eliminate the negative thoughts and feelings and replace them with positive programming. Within months she had let go of the weight she had been carrying and she described feeling better than she had since her kids had been born. She also realized the result of her new beliefs had, in fact been a positive experience for her family as well. They were all more active and eating better as well.

She also felt the experience had set her kids up for success with their own weight and health for the future. She also connected with two women from the neighborhood who had kids of their own. She began to meet up for playdates with her new friends and their children. Sarah reported feeling happier and more settled into her new community than she had since the birth of her children.

Chapter 7

Stan's Story

Stan is a 62-year-old man, who told me he was "ready for a change." When I asked him what he meant, he described his life.

His wife had passed away several years before. Their relationship had been a traditional one, and throughout their marriage Stan had worked long hours and his wife had taken care of the children and the home. They lead a comfortable life, and their social life primarily consisted of time with their children and grandchildren and a small group of married couples that they got together with from time to time.

Stan's wife had always been the "social butterfly" according to Stan and she loved to entertain. Holidays and vacations were times of the year she enjoyed immensely and she planned and hosted parties and dinners at their home throughout the year. She was a much beloved wife, mother and grandmother, and Stan missed her and had felt lost since her passing.

The family had not yet recovered from her loss either. Family occasions were tough, and the family had been drifting away from one another. Nobody knew how to keep the family together, Stan's wife had been the glue and each one of the family members knew something had to change, but nobody knew where to begin.

Even though Stan's wife had been gone four years Stan, had not really figured out how to take care of himself very well. He had a housekeeper who took care of the house, and he was living on fast food and TV dinners. He was lonely as well, and he admitted he was drinking most nights. These new habits had caused Stan to feel sluggish and the extra calories in food and alcohol had caused him to gain 50 pounds.

Stan was clear that he needed to change for himself but, also to help the rest of his family. He had many beliefs that were part of his subconscious programming. Stan and I created a list of programming obstacles that Stan would need to overcome to make changes to his life.

Like many people who want to lose weight, their weight gain can be attributed to specific events in their life. For example, in the case of Sarah, her weight gain was related to the birth of her kids and the family's move to a new town. She had never even thought about what she ate and being physically fit was easier because she did not yet have children, and sports and exercise were part of the social life she shared with her husband and friends.

Stan's weight had been stable throughout his married life and remained so until the death of his wife. Her death brought changes to Stan emotionally, but also caused him to face new challenges such as deciding what to buy and cook, as well as how to get through social events and holidays which had been so special to his late wife.

Stan and I discussed his beliefs about weight and determined that he hadn't really given any thought to what he ate before the death of his wife, as she had been the one making all the decisions about what to buy and how to cook it. Stan realized that it was time to think about the next chapter of his life and he was determined to get control of not just his weight, but the rest of his life.

Stan took almost two weeks to think about what he would need to change in order to gain control of his life. When Stan had determined what was keeping him stuck, it gave us what we needed to create his self-hypnosis script.

As you read Stan's list it may be clear that Stan had a great deal of negative programming that had to be addressed that was not directly related to weight loss. This is not all that unusual. Big changes such as financial upheaval or the death of a loved one can lead directly to weight gain, and addressing these other issues is just as important as dealing directly with weight.

Stan's negative programming

I can't cook.
I don't know how to eat healthy food.
It is not fair that my wife died.
I can't take care of myself.
My life will never be good again.
I am too old to change.
Drinking is the only way I can cope with life.
Cooking is too much work.
Shopping is too confusing.
I can't learn something new.
Exercise is for young people.
My wife always took care of family stuff.
My wife held the family together.
My kids are fine without me.
I hate exercise.
Learning to exercise is too confusing.
Socializing is too much work.

Stan's self-hypnosis script

Induction/relaxation

I close my eyes and let my self sit back, relaxed and comfortable. I imagine I am sitting on a warm sunny beach. It is a beautiful warm day and I feel ready to settle in and to relax. The only sounds are from the warm light breeze, a few birds overhead and the gentle waves that continuously rollup on the shore.

This is a very relaxing place, and it feels so peaceful to come here and take a few moments to relax deeply. This peaceful place is the perfect setting to relax deeply and fully.

I feel the sand warm beneath my feet. My feet and toes sink down a little and a feeling of release in the muscles in my feet and calves comes into this part of my body making me feel so good. The feeling of relaxation spreads up my legs, and my thighs and hips now feel fully relaxed too. I let the muscles be loose, and relaxed.

The feeling of relaxation is one of the best feelings there is. I let my stomach and chest relax. My breath is relaxed and like the waves, it comes in gently and leaves my body gently, each breath relaxes me more. The waves roll in and roll out and I continue down into relaxation, and I let the gentle breeze and the sound of the waves relax me even more.

My arms and shoulders relax now. They feel loose and limp. My neck is so relaxed. All the muscles and fibers go loose, limp, relaxed and my neck muscles release. This great feeling of relaxation spreads up to my jaw and my mouth. I let the muscles be loose, my jaw and face feel relaxed, loose, and limp. The rest of my face feels so relaxed too, the area around my eyes relaxes and the skin and muscles, fibers and every part of my face and neck have let go and I allow them to feel deeply relaxed.

I love this feeling, and as my breath gently moves in and out of my body, I let myself relax and with each breath, and with every gentle wave that washes up on the shore, I relax even more. I am ready for all the wonderful, powerful suggestions I give to myself. They make powerful changes to my subconscious programming and to my life.

Suggestions

Now is the time for me to become unstuck. Like a car that has been stuck in the mud, it is time to let myself pull myself up and out of the mud. I choose now to let myself be unstuck.

Linda was special to me, and I honour her memory. She wants me to be healthy, happy and to have a feeling of freedom about my life. She loved life, she loved our children, and she wants me to keep our beautiful family together. She loved life, our kids and the special occasions and holidays that made this family who we are.

These occasions are important for this family and as the head of this family I choose to make these occasions special once again. I deserve happiness, and a great deal of happiness comes from times spent with my family and close friends. Linda would want this, and I want it too.

I communicate with my children, and we plan ways for the family to rebuild by getting together for family events. We do things together, and it helps build our family and brings us close together once again. I will plan and host some of the special occasions and they will plan and host some of the other ones. I know I will take charge and contact everybody a few weeks before birthdays, or holidays and we will plan together what to do. I want my family to be close again and so I choose to take control. I am a take charge type of person, and I can do this so easily.

I can buy food, I can cook food, I can take the family to a restaurant. We make new traditions and that is ok. Linda would want this, my children want this, and I want this. Family means happiness to me, and I now bring my family close together. I look forward to each family occasion.

Exercise makes my body feel healthy, it helps take off the weight, and relaxes my mind. I have always enjoyed walking and hiking. I get out for a walk seven days each week. I have my fitness tracker which keeps track of my daily steps and calories burned, and I make sure I get my 10,000 steps in every day, and twice a week I will have a longer walk. Walking feels so good, and I release the excess weight on my body.

Getting in my steps every day now is easy. I have many walking trails close to the house. I also ask my grandchildren to go with me for a walk to the park and we walk and run, and I play with them in the playground, and I feel healthy and happy and the pounds melt off my body. It is so easy now. Easier than I thought it would be. The weight melts off and I feel so happy.

I reviewed several eating plans, and I am happy with the choice I made. I have made the decision to learn to cook, by having a meal delivery service become part of how I now eat. The delivery service brings all the ingredients for the meals I have chosen for myself. The food is delivered, and I enjoy this service and it works well for me, as somebody else does the shopping. This helps me become unstuck. I choose my meals for the week, and they deliver what I need. This enables me to begin to understand what I like and what the ingredients are for recipes I enjoy.

The other part about having this service is that each meal I choose has the directions for making the meal. I follow the simple directions and I learn how to cook meals I enjoy, and I am unstuck. I am learning a new skill and I am proud of how I am learning and how I am improving my health. I am proud of myself, and my children and grandchildren are impressed.

The meals also come with a guide which tells me the calories, fat, and protein for each meal. This helps me learn what healthy eating is all about. I am learning and I am proud. I am learning and I am unstuck.

As I become confident with my new cooking skills, I may choose to start shopping for myself as well. My confidence increases and I learn the recipes, and I know the ingredients and I can choose to start doing the grocery shopping for my meals as well. As my confidence grows, I am free to make this choice or perhaps I continue to have my ingredients delivered and then cook my meals following the recipe.

I continue to have my simple breakfast and lunch. Toast and coffee in the morning and a sandwich for lunch. I am confident making these simple meals, and I know what to buy when I go to the store. I shop for these food items, and I feel confident. I also add two pieces of fruit to what I eat during the day. They taste delicious, and they improve my health. I feel full and satisfied by the food I eat during the day. I feel confident about these choices. I improve my health and I am unstuck. I shop for my daytime meals and snacks, and I feel so confident. I am unstuck.

I am unstuck and I connect with my family at least three times per week. I take the time to call them and arrange visits with my family. I take the kids to the park, and I invite them over to share a meal. I like showing off my new cooking skills. We do potlucks, barbeques, and visits to the park. I plan fun things to do with my kids and grandkids. I feel great seeing my kids more and I really love hanging out with my grandkids.

I get to know them, and they get to know me. The family knits itself back together and I help my family rebuild and we are strong and supportive of one another. This makes me feel healthy, and happy and connected. I feel good about my family, and I feel good about myself.

My life is greatly improved with my new plans. I choose to drink less alcohol. I feel better and I drink less. I have more energy. I also sleep better. My confidence grows and my connections to my family are strong. I enjoy this feeling. I drink three times a week or less. I drink two drinks or less each time. I enjoy my life more and more.

It feels good and I enjoy sleeping better and concentrating better and I spend my time with family, and I choose connections over drinking, I choose health instead of drinking. I choose making strong bonds over drinking. I feel better and better, and I am unstuck.

Post-hypnotic suggestions

My beloved wife was a great influence on me and on my family. I know she would want me to be healthy. I know she would want me to be happy. Each time I think about my wife I am aware that she loved me, and she loved our family. I know she would want me to hold this family together and I honour her memory by doing all the things she would want me to be doing.

Each time before I eat a meal, my mind is filled with the thought of my wife, and I imagine her telling me to be strong, and healthy. She reminds me to take care of my health by getting my physical activity and by eating the healthy foods I have chosen for myself. She reminds me to limit the amount of alcohol I take in and to get enough rest each night.

She was the glue that held the family together and, in my mind, I see how well she kept us strong. She reminds me that it is my time now to make sure the family sticks together. She helps me to see how I can plan social events with the family and how I can enjoy my life more by getting out for some fun with the grandchildren. She reminds me that I am now the glue making the family strong, and by helping them stay strong, I am making myself strong and healthy too.

Re-emergence

I have had a great self-hypnosis session today. The suggestions I have given myself make changes to my subconscious mind and change my behaviour.

It is time to re-emerge and get back to my day. I image myself once again on the beach. I feel the warm breeze on my face and hear the waves washing up on the sand.

I begin to emerge by first wiggling my toes, and then lifting my feet and making circles with my ankles. I am starting to feel a bit more awake.

I lift my legs one after the other, and stretch them out in front of me, my body is beginning to feel even more awake.

I lift my arms overhead and move them around, I wiggle my fingers, and shake my arms around, feeling more and more awake.

I open my eyes and stand up. I swing my arms around and march on the spot for 30 seconds and I repeat to myself, "awake, awake, awake."

I move my arms and legs around for another 30 seconds and I repeat to myself, "Wide awake, wide awake, wide awake."

I am now fully awake and ready to get back to my day. I feel energized and excited about all the beneficial changes I am making. I know what to do, and how to do it and it feels so good. I go now and continue with a great day.

Stan's results

Stan reported to me that in the months after our work together that he began to feel like he had turned a corner. He felt healthier, had lost a significant amount of weight, and he had reconnected with his family. He felt like he was a real "grandpa" to his grandchildren which brought him joy every day. He realized that he had reached a dangerous place after the death of his wife, and he knew he was never going to go back to feeling that unhappy ever again.

Stan's success can be your success.

Chapter 8

Jeff's Story

Jeff was 37 years old when we first met. Jeff had been a very successful athlete in his teens, and it had seemed at one time, like he may have a professional hockey career. Unfortunately, he suffered a serious injury which took several months to heal and ended any dreams he had about life as a professional athlete. This was a devastating blow to Jeff, as every part of his life changed after he was injured. The things he had always taken for granted were taken away from him and he found these changes very hard to understand and to cope with.

Fitness had always been important to Jeff. He had been playing hockey and other sports since he was six years old. Having a strong athletic physique had come naturally to him as he spent so much time at hockey practice and playing actual games. He had also been able to eat what he liked and had no need to be careful about portion sizes.

Jeff told me that when he lost his ability to play high level hockey, he really felt lost. His friends and social life had always revolved around hockey, and he really had no other interests or hobbies. He noticed he avoided old friends from his hockey team as it reminded him of what he had lost.

After his injury, Jeff was at first unable to do any exercise at all, and even after his injury had healed, he could no longer play sports, so he never started back into any kind of regular exercise. He also became quite isolated and stayed home on his own for much of the time. He ate a lot of fast food and gained 25 pounds right after he was hurt. He had added another 25 pounds to that initial weight gain, and he reported that he felt terrible, physically, mentally and emotionally.

Jeff was eager to take off the weight and he was also willing to commit himself to self-hypnosis. Jeff understood that the mind is important to success, as he had learned about visualization and positive affirmations from his coaches.

The first thing we did was talk about what he really wanted to accomplish through self-hypnosis. We knew that Jeff could not go back to playing hockey, but he knew he wanted to begin some type of exercise program because he knew how much better he would feel if he exercised. He knew as well that if he began to be physically active, he would lose the extra weight more rapidly.

Jeff described his goals as wanting to lose 50 pounds and find some new ways to get active again. Prior to his injury he was either playing a game of hockey or practicing at least 5 times a week. Jeff wanted to get active again at least 3-5 times a week.

After our initial discussion, Jeff tried a few different sports and exercise programs. He settled on spin classes which are classes with an instructor who leads participants through a workout on stationary bikes. He also began to lift weights three nights a week. He enjoyed these activities and he realized he would enjoy his classes and weight workouts which would help make it easier to maintain his routine.

He also knew how important eating well was to reaching a healthy weight, and he knew that now was the time to actively seek out a new eating program that would be easy to follow, not too difficult to cook, and would leave him feeling satisfied and not feeling hungry all the time.

After a bit of research at a local bookstore, Jeff bought a book
with a reasonable healthy eating plan. His plan included
eating more fruits and vegetables, eating less saturated fats
and giving up quite a bit of the junk food he had been eating.
He felt comfortable with cooking his meals and shopping, so
the plan worked for him. He also decided to take his lunch to
work most days which gave him more control over what he
consumed each day, and as a bonus saved him enough money
to pay for his gym membership.

Jeff knew as well that it was time to start rebuilding a social
life. He had isolated himself to a great degree from his old
hockey teammates and friends and hadn't done anything to
try to meet new people. He knew that if he continued to stay
isolated at home, he would find it much harder to let go of the
extra weight. This is not uncommon. When we are unhappy
and isolated it can be very difficult to motivate ourselves to
change. Having an active family and social life is for most
people strongly connected to improving our chances of losing
excess weight.

Together Jeff and I created a script to help him regain his
health and take off the accumulated pounds.

Jeff's list of negative programming

I was only able to maintain my weight by playing hockey.
I am not sure what exercise I should do now.
My injury keeps me from exercising.
I don't like healthy food.
I don't know what to eat.
Change is too hard.
People see me as a loser.
I am going to be like this forever.

Jeff's negative programming continued.

I will be hungry all the time if I try to diet.
I don't have any friends to socialize with.
It is hard to meet new people.
I find it so hard to meet the right people to date.

Jeff and I worked on a script together which would address his list of goals, and his negative programming. We created suggestions that he would use after reaching his deep relaxed state. Remember affirmations can be helpful to people, but due to the nature of the conscious mind, affirmations may be rejected because the conscious mind can be skeptical. By using one of the scripts that are included at the back of the book, to reach a deep relaxed state, we can bypass the skeptical part of the brain and reach the subconscious mind.

Jeff's script for weight loss and getting in shape

Now that I am resting comfortably with my eyes closed, I take a deep cleansing breath, and I let it out, emptying my lungs completely. I continue to breathe deeply and allow myself to begin to relax.

I imagine myself at the top of a long stone staircase. I take a step down the first step, and I notice I feel safe and calm. I know that the staircase will take me to a calm and peaceful place. I let myself relax even more. I take the next step down and I notice I feel even more relaxed. I continue down the steps and with each step I take, I let myself become more and more relaxed.

I continue to drift down the stairs noticing with each step that I feel more and more relaxed. I enjoy this feeling and I know that in this deep relaxed state I accept the suggestions and they create new programming to my subconscious mind.

I am now becoming very relaxed and if any stray thoughts come into my mind, I notice them, and then let them drift away.

I know that in this deep relaxed state I accept the suggestions I give myself, and they create new programming to my subconscious mind.

I am now very relaxed. I enjoy the feeling of deep relaxation, and now that I am near the bottom of the stairs, I feel so good.

I take the last step now and allow myself to go even more deeply relaxed. In this relaxed state my subconscious mind receives my suggestions and the programming in my subconscious mind changes, and I reach the goals I have set for myself.

I enjoy being physically fit, and I like how it feels to be in shape. I like the feeling of having a strong body. I feel great when I am physically active. I liked that feeling when I was playing hockey and I am excited to get that feeling back. My body looked great when I played hockey. It is time for me to look and feel like I did when I played hockey. That was a good feeling and I have decided now is the time to get that feeling back. I like how good I look when my body is strong and fit. I am taking the time now to get my body in shape.

I think about how my body looks when I am in shape. My arms and chest are strong with defined muscles. My legs and calves are strong and muscular. I take a moment now to think about how great my legs look when I am physical active. My waistline shrinks when I am fit, and my abdominal muscles look strong and defined.

I enjoy healthy food and I know how important it is for my body and mind. I have taken time to seek out a healthy eating plan. I did some research and I have chosen the one that I know works best for me. It is reasonable and healthy.

I have decided to join the gym close to my home. I really enjoy the spin classes and I can work hard, get my heart rate up and have the amazing feeling that a good workout brings me. I do three spin classes each week and then spend 30 minutes doing a weight routine.

 I enjoy my weight program, and my trips to the gym make me feel healthy and energetic. I work out at the same time each day, and I see some of the same people and realize that there are some great people there, and I say hello and chat with people I get to know. I enjoy being social and I like that I have a new way to meet people.

I have also found a group that hikes on the weekends. This group is geared towards singles, and I go and hike with the group every weekend. Friends are important to me, and I like having this opportunity to meet new people. I take time to get to know the other hikers and open my mind to the possibility of making friends.

My new habits feel good, and my body is noticeably slimmer and lighter every week. I notice that my muscles are beginning to develop, and I notice how good they look. These changes make me feel better when I see old friends.

I buy some new clothes which fit me well and make me feel good. I maintain my new lifestyle because I enjoy it and I feel so good. I continue to practice self-hypnosis throughout my life, and it helps me maintain my new healthy strong body.

I change my self-hypnosis routine from time to time when I think I need to, and it makes it easy to keep my body healthy and strong.

Remember to include post-hypnotic suggestions like the ones below, as well as suggestions to leave your deeply relaxed state to the end of every one of your self-hypnosis sessions.

In a few moments I leave this successful self-hypnosis session feeling great. I am about to gradually awaken, knowing my suggestions have reached my subconscious mind enabling me to rewrite any negative programming that may be found there. I know this session was effective and caused changes to my thoughts, beliefs and behaviour. Throughout my day I continue to be aware of these changes and I notice the changes that have been made.

Throughout my day as I move my body, for example when I walk to my car, or exercise or even carry the groceries, I notice that my body feels good, and I feel grateful, positive and energized and my commitment to my new way of life becomes stronger and more powerful. Each time I move my body I become stronger and more energized and happier about my new way of life. This happiness deepens with each movement of my body and my feelings of happiness about the changes I am making become set into new positive habits.

I am now ready to emerge from my hypnotic state. This session has been so good for me. It energized me and I am ready to emerge, and I feel ready for a successful day. In a moment when I count from 10 to 1, each number I say in my mind makes me feel more awake.

10   Now I am ready to emerge and to feel strong and energized.

9   Feeling more awake, livelier and more energized.

8   Now emerging feeling great.

7   Getting ready to start my day more awake and more energized.

6   More energized and more awake.

5   Halfway to being fully awake and fully energized.

4   Almost there, my self-hypnosis is successful.

3   Energized and awake and ready to go back to my day.

2   In a moment when I reach one, I open my eyes, feeling energized, and fully awake.

1   Fully awake now, fully energized for the day. I feel ready for a great day.

Why are post-hypnotic suggestions so important?

This type of suggestion is important because as you go through your day, it enables you to constantly reinforce the new programming you have added to the subconscious mind. Remember we are working to change programming that may be decades old and adding this one small step to your daily practice of self-hypnosis allows the ideas you have presented to your subconscious mind to be strengthened throughout the day.

Post-hypnotic suggestions are presented to the subconscious mind like all other suggestions, while you are in a deeply relaxed state. Post-hypnotic suggestions have two parts. The first part is an action that you perform throughout the day. For example, moving your body, looking in a mirror, or checking your watch or phone. I typically like to use the movement of the body as the first part of my post-hypnotic suggestions because moving our bodies is something we all do often, and it is associated with weight loss goals.

To follow are some examples of post-hypnotic suggestions you can use for your own self-hypnosis practice.

1. As I go through my day, each time I notice a mirror I notice how healthy I look, and I notice how energized I am to reach my goal.

2. Each time I prepare healthy food for myself, a feeling of energy and pride fills my mind and my heart, and I feel more and more energized to reach my goal.

3. When I am involved in physical activity, I become aware of how good my body feels and how much I enjoy being fit and energetic, and I know I want this feeling to stay with me forever.

Remember to always use positive language and use the present tense. That means use phrases such as "I enjoy feeling fit", or "I am energized." Avoid using phrases such as "I **will** feel energized," as it is referring to some unspecified time in the future. When you address your subconscious mind, you must speak like it is something that is already happening. Your subconscious mind does not respond to suggestions given any other way.

Jeff's success can be your success

Jeff had been an athlete for his whole life, and the idea of committing to a plan was something he understood. He felt he had reached a physical and emotional low point, so he was ready to commit himself to beginning his self-hypnosis right away. When he started, he found that he liked to start his day off with self-hypnosis before getting out of bed. He kept his cell phone beside his bed, and as he lived on his own, all he had to do was turn on the recording and listen to it before doing anything else.

Starting your day with self-hypnosis is a great idea. When you have just opened your eyes in the morning you are already in a relaxed state and your mind is ready to accept suggestions. This sleepy state is like the hypnotic state, you are close to sleep yet, you can hear and accept suggestions.

Similarly, the time just before you go to sleep at night is also an excellent time to repeat your self-hypnosis recording. Not only are you in a very relaxed state, so your self-hypnosis will easily reach your subconscious mind, but you will also have the suggestions you have given yourself in your mind as you sleep. This schedule of early morning, and then right before bed is an ideal way to ensure you are getting the full benefit of self-hypnosis.

In addition to listening to his self-hypnosis in the morning and before bed Jeff also took headphones to work with him and found 15 minutes to sit with his eyes closed and listen to his self-hypnosis script. Jeff said he found listening to his self-hypnosis script during the day really motivating. You may choose to do a third session, but that is optional.

Jeff worked in an office, and he had the space to sit back in his chair with his phone and headphones, without being disturbed. He told his co-workers he was taking some time to rest and meditate, and nobody thought it was unusual.

It is easy just to tell people you are resting. You will be in a very deep relaxed state which allows you to make changes to your subconscious mind. You will not be asleep, so if you need to get up or if somebody says something to you, you will hear them. You will be able to simply open your eyes and respond to them.

Jeff's script also included suggestions for coming out of his deeply relaxed state so when he was done, he was wide awake and ready to continue with a productive day. He noted that he felt peaceful and that he felt very refreshed. Jeff enjoyed this short break in his day, as it reduced the stress he sometimes felt in his job. As mentioned earlier, it is not necessary for you to listen to your self-hypnosis script during the day, but it worked well for Jeff.

Jeff began to lose weight right away, and it took him about 8 months to take off the 50 pounds. He also got to know quite a few people from the exercise classes he participated in, and he began getting together with people he met to take classes together and to also do his weight workouts. This led to a new social group and new friendships, which improved Jeff's life significantly.

Jeff has continued to do well and maintain the changes he made. He has reduced the number of self-hypnosis sessions he does daily. He also uses the self-hypnosis skills he learned to help him improve other parts of his life. He uses self-hypnosis as a tool he can use whenever he wants to tweak his diet or exercise programs, or for any other goal he wants to achieve.

Chapter 9

Putting It All Together

There are four parts to a self-hypnosis session. The first part is reaching a deeply relaxed state. The second part is listening to your script of suggestions. The third part is creating post-hypnotic suggestions which will reinforce your programming throughout the day. The fourth part is taking time to emerge from the relaxed state so you can carry on with your day.

Using a cell phone or tablet to record your relaxation script followed directly by your suggestions script is the best way to ensure that the programming in your subconscious mind is changed.

Each self-hypnosis session will begin with an induction which is just another term for putting yourself into a deep state of relaxation where your subconscious mind can be programmed with your new suggestions. I have included inductions throughout the book which you can use and at the back of the book. When you create your own self-hypnosis script, use the induction that works best for you.

While in your deeply relaxed state, the programming suggestions you give yourself will reprogram your subconscious mind. It is also very helpful to include post-hypnotic suggestions which reinforce your subconscious suggestions throughout the day. For example, in Stan's self-hypnosis script, each time he ate a snack or meal, the thought of his wife and what she would have wanted him to do would fill his mind. These suggestions are important, because they help to overcome any negativity that may try to creep in as you go through your day.

Once you have decided which suggestions you will use for your self-hypnosis script, use your cell phone to record the four parts of your script. Recording it will allow you to just get comfortable and listen. This is a very effective way to ensure that you include all the suggestions you have decided will help you meet your goals.

The final part of a self-hypnosis script it the re-emergence. This final part transitions you from being in deep relaxed state to being wide awake and ready to carry on with your day. This part is important so that you feel lively and ready to go to work or carry on with all the activities you need to do throughout the day.

Once you have recorded the four parts of your self-hypnosis script, you are ready to begin to use self-hypnosis to change your life.

All that is left is to find a comfortable place to relax. You could lay down or lay back in a comfortable chair. Start your recording, close your eyes and prepare for all the changes you are creating.

Chapter 10

Scripts For Deep Relaxation

There are many methods that one can use to reach a deep relaxed state where ideas you are repeating can reach your subconscious mind. The method you use is entirely up to you. It works best when you record your relaxation script and your new programming, post-hypnotic suggestions and re-emergence on your phone, so that you can listen to them in sequence, all together.

I have included several relaxation scripts that you can use as is, or you may change them and add your own details.

Elevator script for deep relaxation-shorter version

After finding a quiet comfortable place, take yourself through this script by recording it on your phone and listening to it or by thinking about it in your own mind.

I imagine myself in an elevator; it is quiet in the elevator and I feel calm, safe, and peaceful. I notice a single button with a down arrow on it. I reach out and press the button. Silently, the elevator begins to slowly descend and as it goes farther and farther down, I feel more and more relaxed. I notice I have a feeling of being more and more relaxed and more and more calm and more and more at peace. I am aware that the elevator continues to slowly descend and the further down it goes, the more relaxed I feel. The only sound is my deep calming breaths. It feels good to just let myself go down into relaxion with the elevator. the elevator takes me deeper and deeper down and with every floor I feel myself becoming more peaceful, calmer, and more relaxed.

You are now deeply relaxed and getting more relaxed, the elevator continues to go down and down, and you notice this and feel better as you pass each floor. You notice now with each breath that you take you become more and more relaxed, more and more peaceful and you feel more and more at peace.

You continue to relax until you know it is time to become aware of the new ideas that become important new ideas that cause you to reach your goal. With each breath you notice you are more relaxed, and you are ready to take in these new ideas and in your deep relaxed state the ideas become powerful programming to your subconscious mind.

The elevator gently comes to a stop, and you are calm and peaceful, at ease and deeply relaxed. You are ready for the powerful suggestions that you give to your subconscious mind, so you change your body, mind and spirit.

Total body method for deep relaxation

I am taking the time now to relax and do something great for myself. I relax myself and I feel so good. I take a moment to get nice and comfortable. I make sure the temperature is right for me, I make sure I am laying back in a comfortable position which feels so good.

The first thing I do is tighten every part of my body. I make tight fists; I lift my legs and tighten all the muscles in my feet and legs. I do the same with my arms and hands. I scrunch up my face and my eyes. I take a deep breath and let my whole body relax at once, and as it relaxes, I let it sink down more and more relaxed and each part of my body feels so good.

I think about my feet and legs, and I let all the muscles relax even more, all the muscles go soft and relaxed, and it feels so good. I think about my lower back and my stomach and chest and let those areas go smooth and soft and so relaxed and it feels so good. I check in and make sure my chest feels relaxed, and if I am holding anything there or my breath isn't smooth, I relax it completely, I let it go and it feels so good.

I turn my attention to my neck and my head, and I allow the muscles in my neck and face to relax, go loose and limp and relaxed. It feels good to relax and let go completely and I take a moment now to make sure my whole face, and my head and neck are completely relaxed.

I scan my body, and any area that is not fully relaxed, I relax now. My breath is even, I feel calm and peaceful. It feels so good, and I am ready for all the beneficial suggestions to reach my sub-conscious mind.

Script 2 for deep relaxation

I lay back in a comfortable place. I close my eyes and take a deep breath.

I scan my body and notice if there is any part of it that needs to move to be completely relaxed. I go ahead and move that body part and feel how relaxed it feels. I take a deep breath in and tighten up every muscle in my body, hold that tightness and now I breathe out deeply and let my whole-body flop back and sink deep into relaxation. I turn my attention to my head, and feel how relaxed it feels, I let my face relax, my eyes are closed, my jaw is slack, and all the muscles of my face are smooth.

I notice with each breath that I become more relaxed, each breath takes me another step deeper into relaxation I turn my thoughts gently to my chest and stomach, which are now very deeply related, my breaths are smooth, my muscles are loose, and each breath takes me another step deeper into relaxation and it feels so good.

I am moving into a deep state now. So calm, so peaceful, so relaxed. I move my thoughts gently to my arms and hands. They lay limp and feel heavy, so heavy I don't even want to move them.

My deep breaths continue, and each breath takes me deeper and deeper down and it feels so good. I am going deeper and more relaxed with each breath.

My attention gently turns to my legs and feet, they are loose, calm, relaxed and letting go. They feel calm and heavy, and I let the muscles relax more and more and it feels so good.

I am now completely relaxed, and each breath takes me deeper and deeper, more and more relaxed. This deep state of relaxation feels so good and as each breath takes me deeper.

I begin to think about how deeply relaxed I have become. In this deep state I think about all the changes I am making to my thinking, my feelings and my body.

My subconscious mind receives the new programming easily, the new ideas soak into my subconscious mind easily. They take hold and become rooted there.

These new ideas allow me to make the changes I have been looking forward to. These changes to my thinking, and my beliefs which makes changing my habits and behaviours.

in a simple and natural way.

Beach and waves induction method

I close my eyes and let myself sit back, relaxed and comfortable. I imagine I am sitting on a warm sunny beach. It is a beautiful day warm, and I feel ready to settle in and to relax. The only sounds are from the warm light breeze, a few birds overhead and the gentle waves that continuously rollup on the shore.

This is a very relaxing place, and it feels so peaceful to come here and take a few moments to relax deeply. This peaceful place is the perfect setting to relax deeply and fully.

I feel the sand warm beneath my feet. My feet and toes sink down a little and a feeling of release in the muscles in my feet and calves comes into this part of my body making me feel so good. The feeling of relaxation spreads up my legs, and my thighs and hips now feel fully relaxed too. I let the muscles be loose, and relaxed.

The feeling of relaxation is one of the best feelings there is. I let my stomach and chest relax. My breath is relaxed and like the waves it comes in gently and leaves my body gently, each breath relaxes me more. The waves roll in and roll out and I continue down into relaxation, and I let the gentle breeze and the sound of the waves relax me even more.

My arms and shoulders relax now. They feel loose and limp. My neck is so relaxed. All the muscles and fibers go loose, limp relaxed and my neck muscles release. This great feeling of relaxation spreads up to my jaw and my mouth. I let the muscles be loose, my jaw and face feel relaxed, loose, and limp. The rest of my face feels so relaxed too, the area around my eyes relaxes and the skin and muscles, fibers and every part of my face and neck have let go and I allow them to feel deeply relaxed.

I love this feeling, and as my breath gently moves in and out of my body, I let myself relax and with each breath, and with every gentle wave that washes up on the shore, I relax even more. I am ready for all the wonderful, powerful suggestions I give to myself. They make powerful changes to my subconscious programming and to my life.

Staircase induction method

My mind is ready to listen to all the suggestions about becoming slim and healthy through new ways of eating and new programs of exercise. The suggestions here are powerful and change my body, mind and spirit. I allow myself to take in these suggestions and they enable me to become a success. People become what they believe to be true and that is why it is important to remember to think about how successful I am. Losing weight and eating the foods that will help maintain a healthy slim body is now something that is something I can do. I maintain my habits and the weight stays off.

I am about to allow myself to go to a deeply relaxed state where, the suggestions I give myself are clear and powerful and changes are made to my subconscious mind.

I imagine myself at the top of a beautiful long stone staircase. The details of the railing are beautiful, and the stones beneath my feet are smooth and I am ready to take the first step.

Looking at the staircase makes me feel relaxed and I know that as I travel down the steps, I become more relaxed with each step. I travel down the staircase and each step enables me to become ten times more relaxed. Each step takes me to a deeper state of relaxation.

Slowly, I take the first step down, and I let my relaxation deepen. It feels so good to relax and each step feels more and more relaxing.

I take the second step and I feel more comfortable more relaxed, each step making me ten times more relaxed. Third step now, more relaxed and letting go. Forth step and it feels so good just to let go, and I allow myself to go to an even more deeply relaxed state. The fifth step and I am already so relaxed, but I want to go even deeper, so I take the sixth step and it feels so good just to let go.

Now the seventh step and I am close to being completely relaxed but I want to go even deeper, the more relaxed I am, the better I feel. The eighth step now and I am really enjoying this feeling. I feel dreamy and relaxed, my body is relaxed, and my mind is ready for the powerful suggestions I know will enable me to release the weight I choose to let go of. Now the ninth step, I see it and I take the step knowing how good it feels to be so relaxed. I have reached the tenth and final step and I take the step knowing I am relaxed and ready for the suggestions that change the habits I have chosen to release.

Now that I have reached the bottom of the staircase, I feel relaxed and peaceful and so ready to be a success. In this deep relaxed state, I notice a mirror. It is not a normal mirror which shows how I look, but instead it is a special mirror which shows me how I look at the perfect weight for me.

I see myself at the perfect weight. I notice how my arms look. They look slim and fit. My legs look strong and are the right size for me. They look exactly how I want them to look, and I notice their shape and size, and I notice every detail and those details inspire me to be successful. I also notice my waist and my chest. These areas of my body look just the way I want them to. Slim, fit, the muscles firm and fit. I look strong and healthy.

I notice my neck and my face. My face looks younger and fit and healthy. I look so healthy and confident. My jawline is strong, and I look relaxed and happy. This is a very vivid image, and I can see it. I am so inspired to reach the perfect weight for me, and it makes it so easy to release extra weight.

My imagination is vivid, and I am so ready to receive these new and powerful suggestions. I am a success. I have been successful in so many ways. I know I can achieve anything I set my mind to, and I have decided to set my mind to releasing my excess weight and starting an exercise program. I know this is the most natural thing in the world for me.

In a moment I give myself powerful suggestions which make it easy and pleasant to reach the perfect weight for me.

Fixed object induction

This induction starts with your eyes open, which is different than all the other inductions found in this book. Before starting, find yourself a comfortable place to sit back and relax. Find a spot on the wall somewhere out in front of you and focus your attention upon it.

I focus my attention upon the spot I see on the wall. As I focus my attention upon it, I allow the rest of my body to begin to relax. I let my feet and toes relax, and I let anything I was holding there simply release. My calves relax and I allow the muscles to become loose and limp. My thighs and hips relax, and I let myself sink into my chair and the whole lower part of my body feels so good.

I continue to focus my attention on the spot on the wall and I notice my eyes are beginning to feel tired and heavy but still I continue to focus on the spot I see before me. I know my eyes are about to droop, become heavy and close.

I let my stomach and chest relax and my breathing is calm and steady, and each breath relaxes me more and more. I am letting my body become loose, relaxed, and filled with peace and it feels good.

I continue to focus on the spot on the wall, but I notice my eyelids are growing heavy and I want to shut my eyes, it feels so good to let them finally release. My eyelids droop down, and I close my eyes and it deepens my relaxation more and more.

My body continues to relax, and I let my hands and arms become relaxed, I could raise my hands if I wanted to, but they feel heavy now and I just simply let them sink down and down into deeper relaxation.

I let my shoulders and neck let go, and the muscles are loose, relaxed and it feels so good. I allow my jaw to relax and hang slack and all the muscles around my mouth relax too. Letting go more and more and my eyelids feel even heavier. I let all the muscles around my eyes and in my face go completely loose now.

I am relaxed and ready for all the beneficial suggestions I give my subconscious mind. These suggestions change my body mind and spirit and I reach my goals and I feel so good.

Drain away your stress induction

Find yourself a comfortable place to sit back and relax. Close your eyes and imagine that you can simply drain away any tension you have in your body and that these feelings are going to drain away through your fingers and your toes.

Turn your attention to your head and your face, let anything that is interfering with complete relaxation drain down into your neck and down through your body. Your head feels relaxed, and the muscles around your eyes and in your jaw are free to hang loose and limp and it feels good to let go.

Let those feelings, and anything you have been holding on to drain downward. Let your shoulders and your upper back relax, and the muscles there lie smooth and peaceful. And everything else simply drains down through your upper arms, draining down into your lower arms and wrists. Relaxation floods in, and anything you may have been holding on to, now drains out of your fingertips and you let it go. All that is left in your upper body is relaxation as you let go, loose and limp.

Focus for a moment on your chest. Take a nice deep breath in and slowly release it, and anything there that needs to be release, begins to drain down through your body to be released through your toes. All that is left in your chest is full and complete peace and relaxation. Now let your stomach and hips relax and the muscles are free to smooth out and it feels so good.

Your thighs relax and anything you held onto begins to drain down and your thighs are relaxed. Your knees relax and your calves.

As anything keeping you from relaxing drains down and leaves through your fingertips and toes, you feel amazing. Relaxed, peaceful, and letting yourself completely let go. Anything you were holding on to, you let go of now. Take a moment now, to check to see if you are fully relaxed and just let go of anything else.

You are now ready for the powerful suggestions you provide to your subconscious mind to take full effect and they change your thoughts, and behaviours and you succeed in reaching your goals.

Post-hypnotic suggestions

Along with the suggestions you are creating for yourself, I also recommend you add post-hypnotic suggestions to your self-hypnosis script. Post-hypnotic suggestions are suggestions that remind you throughout the day what your goals are. They also reinforce your new programming.

Post-hypnotic suggestions are typically linked to things we de often throughout the day. For example, you may prepare meals several times a day and a post-hypnotic suggestion would be linked to times you are engaged in that activity.

Examples of post-hypnotic suggestions you may use:

1. Each time I look in a mirror I notice how healthy I look, and I notice how energized I am to reach my goal.

2. Each time I prepare healthy food for myself, a feeling of energy and pride fills my mind and my heart, and I feel more and more energized to reach my goal.

3. When I am involved in physical activity, I become aware of how good my body feels and how much I enjoy being fit and energetic, and I know I want this feeling to stay with me forever.

4. Throughout my day as I move my body, for example when I walk to my car, or exercise or even carry the groceries, I notice that my body feels good, and I feel grateful, positive, and energized and my commitment to my new way of life becomes stronger and more powerful.

5. I know how great I look at the perfect weight for me. Each time I eat a meal or a snack, the image of myself at the perfect weight for me, fills my mind and energizes me to continue with all the changes I have made. I take a moment to see that image clearly in my mind. I see my face, slim and bright, and healthy. I see my neck and my chest and my arms. They look strong and fit, and they look great at the perfect size and shape for me.

Chapter 11

Putting it all together

Now is the time to start creating your own script for making all the changes you have been thinking about for so long. There are four steps to creating your script. I will list them here along with a brief description. It is best to record them on a phone or another recording device so that you can find a comfortable spot to relax with your eyes closed.

Part 1: Induction

During the induction, you take yourself to a deep state of relaxation. This part is so important, because it enables the suggestions to by-pass the naturally skeptical conscious mind. Be sure to stay awake during the induction so that you hear all the suggestions.

Part 2: Suggestions

During this part, you give yourself the powerful suggestions that you have created. The suggestions are based upon your list of negative programming. For example, if you have listened for ages about how women always gain weight as they get older, you must change the negative to a positive such as "just because my mom gained weight as she aged, it doesn't mean that will be my story."

Part 3: Post-hypnotic suggestions

Post-hypnotic suggestions are the third part of your self-hypnosis script. This type of suggestion is tied to activities you do throughout the day. For example, "each time I exercise, I

Part 3: Post-hypnotic suggestions

Post-hypnotic suggestions are the third part of your self-hypnosis script. This type of suggestion is tied to activities you do throughout the day. For example, "each time I exercise, I notice how great my body looks and feels and I want to have this feeling every day." These suggestions help to remind your subconscious mind about what your goals are and keep you feeling strong and energized.

Part 4: Re-emergence

In this part of your session, you will move from your deeply relaxed state to a state of full wakefulness. It is important to re-emerge completely so that you can be ready for the rest of your day. Typically, you give yourself suggestions that help energize your mind, and you also begin to gently move your body until you feel wide awake.

How to change your negative programming into positive suggestions

Once you have spent some time thinking about the negative programming that is holding you back, it is time to begin to create a self-hypnosis script to help you successfully lose weight and get into shape. Your self-hypnosis script is personal but, you can of course use any of the scripts found in this book.

It is important to do your best to unearth as many of the negative beliefs you have, and for each of those beliefs, create a positive suggestion. Let's look at a few common negative beliefs that keep people from taking off weight and getting into shape.

Changing Negatives into Positives

Negative Belief	Positive Suggestions
I come from an overweight family, I am just like my family, we have always been heavy.	I am completely different from my family, I am choosing a new way to live, not everybody is heavy in my family.
I hate exercise, exercise is too hard, I don't know how to start an exercise program.	I seek out different types of exercise and choose one I like. Being overweight and out of shape is hard and exercise makes my life so much easier.
My family won't like me if I lose weight. Family gatherings will be too hard. I always overeat at family gatherings.	My family loves me, and I love them, I ask them to support me, and I continue to enjoy our time together, I simply eat a little less.
I must cook for the family, and they don't like healthy food. My kids are too picky to eat better.	I find ways to eat healthy foods that the whole family enjoys, my whole family benefits from the new healthy choices we make, I am setting my family up for success with their own health in the future.
People make fun of me when I eat rabbit food, it is embarrassing to diet.	Lots of people eat in different ways, some people are vegetarian, some are gluten free. I am an adult and I have a right to eat what I like, and I ask people to support me in my efforts to be healthy.
My partner or spouse always did all the cooking. I don't know how to cook. Learning to cook is too hard.	Life changes and that is ok. I find new ways to live and new ways to eat. I can read books, take a cooking class, and talk to friends. I am a strong capable adult and I make changes to my life that benefit me and those around me.

Conclusion

The power of your own mind has kept you from making changes to your eating habits and your ability to reduce your weight. Your beliefs have kept you from finding an exercise program you enjoy and that you will be able to sustain for a long period of time. Now that you have read this book you know what you can do to change your thoughts, your beliefs and habits.

I know a lot of the information is new to you. You may have never thought too much about why you behave the way you do. That is ok. However, if you have been unsuccessful in the past, and you have tried diets and exercise programs in the past, perhaps trying something new is just what you need.

I have spoken to many people who are just like you, desperate for change and out of ideas. People who have tried and failed many times. I always tell them the same thing which is; if your beliefs tell you losing weight and getting in shape is impossible, there is no way to succeed, and will power alone is not enough to overcome powerful subconscious programming.

Make a commitment to yourself to make changes to your beliefs by using the techniques you have learned here. Think about your own negative beliefs, create new positive programming and see the changes to your habits. I have seen the power of the subconscious mind in my own life, and I have seen it work for others and I know it can work for you.

9 798542 969282